INTRUDER

Naturally Kicking Cancer Out

RESCHELLE MEANS

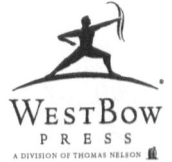

WESTBOW
P R E S S
A DIVISION OF THOMAS NELSON

WestBow Press books may be ordered through booksellers or by contacting:

WestBow Press
A Division of Thomas Nelson
1663 Liberty Drive
Bloomington, IN 47403
www.westbowpress.com
1-(866) 928-1240

ISBN: 978-1-4497-1841-1 (sc)
ISBN: 978-1-4497-1843-5 (hc)
ISBN: 978-1-4497-1842-8 (e)

Library of Congress Control Number: 2011929737

Printed in the United States of America

WestBow Press rev. date: 09/23/2011

CONTENTS

ACKNOWLEDGEMENTS

First and for most I'd like to thank the Father of all creations, who loved me so graciously and endlessly that He chose me for such a time and an assignment as this. I'm ever so grateful. Thank you for Your grace that supplied my every need during my time of trial. Lord this is Your story I'm so grateful that You allowed me to live it and share it. You are my one true heart's desire!

To my loving husband Aubrey who God used to take care of me, provide and protect me through this trying ordeal. I praise God for your love and your support. You ministered to me in ways that I can't explain. When I needed direction and couldn't hear God, He spoke through you at times. You are forever loved and so wonderfully appreciated. You never complained not once when things got rough or expensive. God is so awesome not just anyone could have been in my life, but God knew just who and what I needed for the journey that awaited us me. I love you sweetheart!

To my family; my sisters Kalisha and Jamila (My Precious Critter Bug), my mother Hattie, my aunt Shelia and my brothers Xavier, Jonathan, Todd and Quane; I really appreciate all of you guys support. I know that if it wasn't for you all, I wouldn't be nowhere near where I am today. We have banned together as a family through prayer, studying and researching the changes we all could make, and move toward better health. Thank you again and I love you all.

To my friends Roxanne, Hattie, Kerri, Bonita, Quilla , Tawanna (My Poo Bear), Angie (Queen Geter), First lady Reva and to all those in the Primerica No limit Soldiers Base shop, in Greenville SC you guys rock! Thank you guys so much for all the prayers, the kind words, the phone calls and your genuine concern. I see your hearts and praise God for you.

Last of all, I want to thank the doctors because if it wasn't' for what you all didn't tell me; I may have never went in the opposite direction.

ISAIAH 53:4, 5

Surely He has borne our grief's and carried our sorrows; Yet we esteemed Him stricken, Smitten by God, and afflicted But He was wounded for our transgressions, He was bruised for our iniquities: The chastisement for our peace was upon Him and by His stripes we are healed.

INTRODUCTION

Are you one of those people who has always heard and read about the healing Power of God? You've read in the bible where Jesus healed many that were sick, but in this day and time you feel that it's unheard of. You know that He can do all things, but you have never experienced His supernatural healing power yourself. If you're not sure about who God is, this book will reveal to you His nature, and the keys to experiencing His supernatural power for yourself. I urge you to sit back, grab a cup of hot green tea and get comfortable. Take a journey with me through my life and pay special attention to the up and down struggle as I was persistent in pursuing divine health. You will see the word of God in demonstration and His healing power released in the earth.

This book is intended to educate and inform you of the dangers of trusting in man, and not in God. Through the things that God has allowed me to encounter, I have come to realize that suffering has its place in life. God uses it as a tool to prune us, and produce fruit that would never surface, had not we encountered the pain and the suffering that we experienced. Even though sickness is not of God, God allowed it. This book is not intended to persuade or influence you in any way. If you or someone you know is suffering from an illness, seek professional help. God works through doctors, nurses and medicine also. However it's according to your faith that you are made whole.

CHAPTER 1

How it All Began

My life before now was constant. I felt that there was always something that needed to be done; at least that's how I felt at the time. I'm explaining my life starting from December 2009. Christmas was always my favorite time of the year, except for my birthday of course. As I was preparing my home for the holidays and finishing up the semester in school; I was looking forward to a cheerful Holiday and a new year full of great expectations. Things began to turn around quickly. One day I received a call from my sister telling me she was taking our mother to the ER due to pains in her stomach.

I remember dropping everything and rushing to the hospital. By the time I had gotten there the doctors were running a series of tests to see what the problem was. Besides me and my brothers and sister being born, I had never known our mom to be in the hospital for anything. So this was an alarming time for my family and I. After the results came in from the tests that she had taken, the doctor walked in and told us my mother had a bad gall bladder and that it needed to be removed. The concern was that her gall bladder was not only bad but it was surrounded by what the doctor described as a "swarm of veins".

The risks concerning the operation were, the veins were huge and with so many it was possible that the doctors could cut one by accident and she would bleed to death. My family was frantic, and needless to say, so was I. We didn't know what to think. All we could do was pray and ask God to let it be alright. My mother was transferred to Greenville Memorial, because the hospital had never seen a situation like this. She was admitted and they continued to run more tests. It was as if the doctors were spinning their wheels trying to figure out how to approach the situation.

My family and I came together in prayer, as we believed God would work it out. I don't know if you've ever experienced how stressful hospitals can be, but I became stressed and didn't really realize it after spending days and long hours there. While my family remained at the hospital, I managed to complete all of my exams and pass all of my classes, by the strength of God. It seemed as if the hours and days were getting longer while we waited to see what approach the doctors were going to take. The wait became unbearable at times.

Nothing seemed to change. The doctors still didn't know what to think as we became more concerned. We leaned on each other and the healing power of God to get us through. My mother stayed in the hospital for about four days and was released without surgery or anything, just a lot of tests. They did however give her some pain medicine as they released her, and she felt better for awhile. Christmas by this time was a few weeks away. That year I decided to go all out and pick up just about everyone I knew a gift. I don't know what I was thinking, especially with so much already going on.

Even though my mother was out of the hospital, I remained stressed without much sleep, but felt compelled to keep going. I had so much to get done and so little time to do it in. My mind and body were going on fumes. I was in a place, and wondered how I had gotten there. There were dinner parties my husband and I attended in the evenings. I've always been the type of person who enjoyed relaxing at home. So to be constantly on the move was a lot for me. My body continued to show signs of stress that I had never experienced before.

In all the business I began to neglect my personal relationship with God. The week before Christmas my husband and I had something planned every day of the week except that Saturday. I had planned on taking that day to rest. There was one thing I had been holding back from my husband; I had been having pains in my chest for three days. I couldn't take the pain anymore and finally told him, and he immediately took me to the ER. I was seen rather quickly because chest pains are considered to be more serious than some of the other emergencies.

The doctors took blood, some x-rays and did an EKG; everything came back normal. He asked me what had been going on in my life. I told him and he suggested that I was under a great amount of stress. He said that stress can cause pain in the chest wall, and I should try to take it easy for awhile, and take Ibuprofen. With very little rest that evening; my husband and I headed out to Florida the next morning. We stayed there for four days. We had a good time, but the hustle and bustle of traveling and adventure while I was in Florida didn't make my situation any better.

One thing good did come out of the trip though; my in-laws and I had a chance to get to know each other better. I was still a new wife at that time, and hadn't come to know his family on a personal level. We cooked for each other, played games and just had a wonderful time. I tried to ignore the weariness I felt, because I had every intention on enjoying myself with my new family. If you please continue reading you will see how everything I went through played a huge part in what happened in my life.

We made it back from Florida safely praise God and by the time the New Year approached, I was looking forward to some rest and all the fullness that the year would bring. We celebrated my husband's 39th birthday with dinner and friends. A couple of days later my mother went back into the hospital from constant pain in her side. We knew it had to be her gall bladder since the doctors never did anything about it the first time. She left from work and drove herself to the hospital, and once again transferred back to the same hospital. I began to relive her first experience all over again.

They gave us the decision to drive her to Greenville Memorial or transport her through ambulance. I drove her there and she received a bed very quickly. I think I stayed with her until 10:00 that night. My mother was extremely exhausted, so I decided to leave and let her get a good night sleep. Sometime over in the night the doctors came in her room, and told her they were doing surgery on her early that morning. I'm sure she was scared at the time and it alarmed all of us when we got there. Anyway, to make a long story short she had the surgery and it was a great success Praise God!

CHAPTER 2

What a Way to Start the New Year

We continued to stay at the hospital with her until she was released and went home. My brothers, and sister, and I all assisted in taking care of our mom during her recovery. By this time it was around January 12th. My husband and I were leaving for a fast start school in Winston Salem on the 15th; that's where my journey really began. Little did I know what awaited me was nothing more than what seemed like a nightmare that I couldn't wake up from. I thought for sure everything was good by now, since my mother had her surgery and was doing well. As long as she was ok, I felt I could handle anything else that came my way.

The drive to Winston Salem was nice and peaceful, so I dozed off once or twice. We started out kind of late and arrived around 6 pm Friday evening. We had just enough time to get our bags up to the room and get unpacked before my husband would head down stairs to his meeting, along with the other Regional Vice Presidents from the surrounding areas.

I stayed in the room while he went to his meeting, and found it be relaxing. I was in a different environment and had no plans except to unwind that evening. I remember lying around watching television, talking with my family and friends on the phone, and doing some work on my computer. My evening was perfect. As the hour got late I went to take a shower. As I was washing I felt some tenderness in my right thigh. I remember thinking to myself, *what in the world is this?* As I touched it, I felt a small knot.

I continued to bathe but thought about it all night. When my husband returned, I told him of my discovery. He could see that I was very concerned and said when we get home we would go and have the doctor check it out. Even though he said we would have it checked out, I still don't believe he took me seriously. He told me later that he thought it probably came from me being clumsy around the house. He thought that maybe I had run into a dresser or something, as I usually did from time to time. I continued to monitor it over the next couple of days, but it never went away.

We continued our weekend in Winston Salem and had a wonderful time. When we got back home, I went to the doctor about a week later. I praise God for being all knowing, because I had just gotten health insurance on January 4th. The insurance company called me out of the blue; asking me about purchasing insurance. I knew I needed it, but hadn't gotten around to getting it. I'm painting you a picture to show you how God had things already set up. I had no idea at the time the insurance was going to be much needed.

From One Doctor to Another

I initially went to my family doctor who after poking his finger into my thigh and pressing down on the knot thought it was a small cyst, but couldn't be sure. He then made an appointment for me to have x-rays done. As I had the x-rays done, I thought it was a little strange that the technician was standing behind a glass wall. Little did I know at that time he was protecting himself from the radiation. I had to lay flat on my back as beams of radiation would flow through my body. The results came back and showed "a bunch of tissues", as the nurse called it, but couldn't be sure as to what it was.

In all of this, I remember thinking, *"Wow this sounds kind of serious"* because in the next couple of days my husband and I would be returning back to a different doctor for the third time, and this time it was with a surgeon. I tried to stay focused and told myself not to worry, because I knew God was with me. The doctor had me undress as he pressed his finger into the knot. By this time, the knot had gotten bigger and tenderer. The doctor suggested that it was a lymph node, and stated that it was possible that lymph nodes would go away with an antibiotic.

He wrote me a ten-day prescription to see if the lymph node would dissolve. If not, he said the next step would be surgery, followed by a biopsy. By this time I'm thinking, *"What surgery? And a biopsy are you serious!"* I hate needles, and all I could think about was the anesthesia. I had all kinds of thoughts going through my mind by this time. For some strange reason, and maybe I had been watching too much television, I was worried that when I was under the medication, the doctors would try and take advantage of me. I know, silly thinking right? I told you I had all kinds of thoughts going through my head.

At that point, my mind had gotten the best of me. After all, I hadn't even tried the prescription to see if was going to remove the node. I had to encourage myself and pull it together. I got the prescription filled and took it for ten days as directed. I continued to go to school every day as I took the medicine and was sure that it would do what it was prescribed to do, which was dissolve the lymph node. I prayed and asked God to cover me. Well sure enough, after the ten days was up the lymph node had gotten smaller, but it was still there.

Since the lymph node was still there, I knew the next step was surgery. It took me awhile to digest going under the knife. I had never had surgery before, and frankly I was very afraid. Through prayer and allowing God to do what He needed to do in me; when the time came for surgery on the morning of March 4, 2010, God had wrapped me up in His peace. I felt the assurance that all was going to be well. I would remind myself *"He that dwelled in the secret place of the most high shall abide under the shadow of the almighty."* (Ps. 91:1) God's Word gave me comfort.

My husband was right there to see me through as I faced having surgery. The nurse called me back as she began to prepare me mentally about the procedure, and what all else would take place. When I woke up, my family and my friend Hattie was there waiting with my husband. I couldn't believe that I had the surgery because I wasn't in any pain, but I remembered being extremely sleepy from the medicine. A biopsy was immediately performed. Little did I know, while I was under the anesthesia the doctors told my family that the lymph node looked very suspicious.

My family kept this from me, because they didn't want to upset me, and I could understand why. I had to wait a week and a half for the biopsy report to come back. My faith was really being tested at this point because it seemed as if it took forever for the results to come back. As the days went by, there was still no pain. I had to remove the bandage to see the scar, to remind myself that I had the surgery because I felt completely fine. It was unbelievable because I had this huge scar on my thigh, and it was evident that I had the surgery, but felt absolutely no pain. Now all my family and I could do was wait and pray as the results came back.

I called the doctor's office about four times, and each time a different nurse gave me a different story as to why my results weren't in. I was told it would be around three to four days before the results were in and here it was around the fifth and sixth day. I became very anxious and I started to think there must be something seriously wrong since the doctor hadn't called me. Fear gripped me, as I tried to hold on to my faith. Finally, the nurse called me one morning about 8:00 and asked my husband and I to come in around noon. I became very concerned because I didn't know what the doctors were going to tell me.

CHAPTER 3

The Moment of Truth

I figured the news must not have been good, because the doctor had previously told me if it was nothing to worry about, he would tell me the results over the phone. He said if it was more serious, I would have to come in and he would tell me in person. As we sat there waiting to be called back, I can't describe to you the tension and nervousness I felt. When they called me back, my husband, mother, and sister were with me. The doctor came in the room and said very calmly, *"You have Hodgkin's disease which is a type of cancer."*

I asked the doctor, *"What is Hodgkin's disease?"* I was under the impression it was something that older people got. Well to my surprise, it was a type of cancer that attacks the lymphatic system, and it can show up in young women and men in their twenties and thirties. The doctor had this look on his face as if it was so hard to break the news to my family and I. I wanted to be sure I heard the doctor correctly so I asked *"Are you saying that I have cancer?"* The doctor said, *"Yes."* If I didn't know God was real, I knew He was when the report came in, because the power of God kept me in that moment. However, I was in a state of shock as I had to digest what was being said to me.

My mind went into process mode as my family began to ask different questions concerning the report. Dr. Tate was the surgeon, who I considered to be a good doctor, and very calm as he tried to explain in detail the diagnosis. My mother immediately said *"I rebuke that in the name of Jesus!"* My husband stood calmly, listening very careful as the doctor explained the disease. When the doctor walked out of the room, my sister looked up Hodgkin's disease on her iPhone and told us the disease has a very high survival rate.

One of the nurses walked in as the doctor walked out and said to us, *"Out of all the cancer's, Hodgkin's is one of the most curable one's out there."* She said if a person just had to have cancer, this is the one to have, because it's not only treatable but curable. That was refreshing to hear, but to me at that time cancer was still cancer, and I didn't want to have anything to do with it. My husband and family were a great support and from that moment on we prayed and asked God to show us the way. I think my family felt great sadness for me as well as hope because of the survival rate.

As we left the surgeon's, we stopped on the way out to schedule an appointment with the cancer center. When we got outside, my husband immediately called his mother and told her the diagnosis. In that moment, he expressed his great sorrow and hurt. On the way home we drove in complete silence; it was as if we both were numb and couldn't speak. The word *intruder* kept ringing in my spirit. At the time, I still didn't get it because of everything that had just happened.

Lord, I Need You

As things became clearer, I heard the words invasion of privacy. I began to rationalize in my mind that somehow I had left the door open for the enemy to walk right in. As the days turned to weeks; I continued to examine myself. I went over and over in my head, asking myself what caused this? Was it something I ate, or drank? Was it something I did or didn't do? Needless to say, I was at a place that only God could help me, so I turned to Him and began to confess sin that was in my life. In my mind, I just wanted to be right with God, because I needed Him now more than I ever did.

God is a holy God, and in order to come before Him, you must confess any sins and come clean with Him. I needed the pathway to be clear; I needed the heavens to open up on my behalf, so I was willing to do whatever it took to get into His presence. The ultimate fight for my life had begun. I even started repenting for other people's sin. I was desperate. It wasn't that I was so out of line or playing with sin. It was I had been so distracted by everything that had previously gone on in my life; I began to neglect my relationship with God. I wasn't praying and studying as I normally had been. Thus I was caught off guard.

I didn't want to believe sickness was of God. Nevertheless, God allowed this affliction, so it must have been for a good reason. I wasn't mad at God; I just knew it was something that my family and I were going to have to deal with. As days went by I grabbed a hold of God's extended hand, and I chose to walk closer and put all my trust in Him. I heard the diagnosis but didn't accept it. I grew up in a household where sickness was not accepted. Maybe it was because my mother worked in the healthcare field and worked around sick people all day. When she came home from work, she didn't want to see anymore sickness. So whatever ache or pain we had, we had better be over it by the time she came home. This seems like a cold and heartless attitude to have but, that's how I was brought up had a lot to do with my mindset concerning sickness. My mother wouldn't accept it and neither was I.

I remember when I got home from the doctor's office the internet was down, which was strange. I wanted to research Hodgkin's disease and see what all it entails. It took about four days for the internet to come back up, so one day I went to the office and got on the computer and began to research Hodgkin's, as I would researched anything. I should have never done that. God allowed that internet to be down for a reason. By the time I got off the computer, I was a mess. I read some things online that really scared me and needless to say I was filled with fear. My husband saw me on the computer, and knew exactly what I was doing so he suggested that I get off the computer. Because of the fear, I needed to think, and honestly I didn't know what I was going to do.

CHAPTER 4

There Is Hope

So I drove to the park; a place I could go to think and pray. It was my place of refuge and safety. When I got there, I sat in my car and cried out to God. I cried out over and over, *"No, Lord please this can't be happening!"* After about forty five minutes of sobbing; all of a sudden my tears dried up, and I felt the peace of God like never before. The Holy Spirit prompted me to call a good friend of mine. I called First Lady Reva and began to explain to her the doctor's report. She immediately told me what to do. She told me her mom had been diagnosed with stage four cancer, and they began to treat her with natural and herbal supplements.

She suggested that I purchase some barley powder, Japanese mushroom vitamins, and aloe vera juice from the Whole Food Store. She also told me they prayed over her mom day in and day out. They would anoint her daily, and made sure the Word of God was being deposited into her spirit. I felt so much better because I knew there was something I could do. I went back to my husband's office, and he noticed right off that my attitude was different. He heard hope in my voice. I told him what First Lady had told me, and that I was going to the store to purchase the items she suggested.

When I got to the Whole Food Store, I asked a guy in the store, *"What is good to take if the doctor says someone has cancer?"* This guy referred me to a woman named Lorena. I asked her the same question. She asked me, *"Who has cancer?"* I told her, *"The doctors say that I have it."* I want to pause right here to say since you are reading this book, notice that I say *"they say"* I have cancer. Never claim something you don't want. The cancer wasn't mine and I was not about to claim it. Anyway as I was saying; she suggested barley powder, aloe vera, mushroom vitamins and some other things. Everything she suggested was on the list that First Lady Reva suggested. I knew right then, I was in the right place, at the right time, buying the right things, glory to God!

Lorena also told me she was diagnosed with Thyroid cancer about ten years earlier, and that she refused chemo, surgery, and radiation, and there was no cancer in her system. I'm thinking to myself, *"What?"* I couldn't believe that God had led me to a person who was able to defeat cancer without the standard treatments of chemo and radiation. I felt even more empowered. I had God on my side and now some proof; there were other ways cancer could be cured. She said she started treating herself with natural herbs and supplements, as she changed her diet. She introduced me to this website called Hallelujah Acers; it was a website about raw foods. I began to search through this website, and learned how to prepare meals and the importance of eating the right foods. Lorena and another employee named Mike were extremely helpful. I had so many questions, and for every question, they had an answer.

I got all the things that were suggested. When I left the Whole Food Store, I had spent about seventy dollars, and walked out with one small bag. It was crazy, but that was the best seventy dollars I had ever spent. It was there, I learned if I had been exercising, eating right, and drinking plenty of water, I could have alleviated the lymph node in the first place. I was advised to cut out all sugar, and was told that sugar and cancer feed on each other. These were all the things I felt the doctors should have told me immediately.

I felt they were only interested in the disease and not my personal well being. I wanted to know how I could get well, but really wasn't getting the answers that I needed. Along with the supplements, I was advised to go on a raw food diet. At first I didn't understand how anyone could eat raw foods. It took me awhile before I started with the raw foods, but I did immediately cut all sugars, sodas, bread, fried foods, and basically all meat except baked chicken. This was by no means easy, but for the sake of my health, I couldn't think twice about it.

Now with the biggest part of my meals being cut out, I began to lose weight very quickly. Instead of me feeling worse, because of the cancer; I actually started feeling better. My skin became clearer, I started to feel healthier and stronger than I had ever felt. Once I stopped eating sugar, I didn't feel as weighed down and bloated. My diet was horrible but I was able to see immediate changes in my body once I corrected that.

I also became obsessed with reading God's Word. I continued to search the scriptures on healing and the promises of God started to come alive, as my body was going through transition. God's word alone gives life and provides empowerments.

Finally time had come for my first visit at the cancer center. When I got there the oncologist had my biopsy reports, and had me scheduled right away for bone marrow testing. After listening to the doctors my husband asked the question; *"What does she need to do differently? Does she need to change her diet or anything to help herself get well?"* The oncologist exact words were; *"Oh no, she can continue to eat what she has been eating, because with this type of cancer, it doesn't matter what she eats."* I knew right then and there that I couldn't trust the doctors. I couldn't figure out why he would tell me that. I already knew what they were telling me from the Whole Food store about my diet, so I felt for sure the doctor would back up at least that part, and confirm that I did need to change my eating habits.

The oncologist gave me no advice as to how I could help myself get well. The more I talked with people, and the more I began to research I saw that there were all sorts of things I could have done differently, and could still do to get well. At first I really thought the doctors were trying to kill me. The treatments they would use would keep me sick, and thus expenses would be at an all time high. I felt they were offering treatments that couldn't guarantee a great outcome. It didn't take me long to figure out it was all about the money.

I had to lay aside all of my previous assumptions about how I ate, and took care of myself and start all over. I was at a point where everything I thought was right was actually wrong, and I needed God to show me how to take care of myself. I realized the body was designed to heal itself, but it would take a lot of discipline and a strong will. My oncologist then suggested that I do five weeks of radiation, five days a week. My husband and I thought at the time; at least it wasn't chemotherapy.

Since they said the cancer was in my lymph nodes, they wanted to be sure it hadn't traveled into my bones and spleen. I don't know if you've ever had a bone marrow test done or not, or maybe you know of someone who has, but that is the most excruciating pain I had ever been in. The test is actually worse than the surgery. I was sore for two days, and the whole time the test was being done, I cried. My husband was great, he stood by my side holding my hand, and encouraging me as he watched the oncologist drill me in the back with this very long needle.

The oncologist was a short man, so he had to stand up over me on a stool as he dug into my back to get the marrow. I was given a very painful shot that was supposed to numb me, so I wouldn't feel it when he got the marrow out. Needless to say, I felt way more than I was supposed to feel. The oncologist told me I had strong bones so he had to apply three times the pressure into my lower back as he dug deeper and deeper. All the while a nurse was standing by wiping the sweat off his forehead. Finally he got it after about twenty minutes, praise God. The pain from the procedure caused tears to stream down my face all the way home.

I wasn't able to walk. My husband had to get me up the stairs, and all I could do for the next day and a half was stay in bed. My husband is so precious. He had a big meeting that night at work, with a lot of new people joining him in business. I insisted that he go and have his meeting ,and that I would be okay. I stayed in bed and slept the rest of the evening. I could tell he hated leaving me because of his hesitation, and within two hours he was finished and came home to finish taking care of me.

I was scheduled a couple of weeks out to have a PET and CT scan done. The purpose of the scans was to see how far the cancer had spread throughout my body. As I waited for the time to have the scans to done; I continued to focus on eating right and making sure I had the right mindset. I was very hopeful that if I did everything I was supposed to do, by the time I take the tests no cancer would show up. I was on an all out prow, seeking and researching everything I could get my hands on. I was so determined that this cancer was getting out of my body.

Faith Activated

I started sowing seeds into Dr. Mike Murdock's ministry, and sowed anywhere else I felt led to sow. I encourage you if you're believing God for healing, activate your faith. Look for ways and opportunities to sow seeds. The principle of sowing and reaping doesn't fail. If you sow, you will reap. God's Word doesn't lie. I was faithful taking my supplements, along with drinking plenty of water and exercise. I felt really good about everything I was doing.

People kept coming up to me telling me all kinds of stories about loved ones who had died from cancer. One lady told me she lost three friends to breast cancer in one year; while another person told me he had lost two cousins. I tell you, I basically heard no survival stories, and it seemed like death was all around. Everyone knew someone who had died of cancer. I don't fault anyone for sharing with me, but I had to listen and not hear. I couldn't allow my mind to focus on death. Most people who hear the word cancer immediately think it's a death sentence. I guarantee you will hear other stories. It's a given. Just don't let that cause you to be frighten and lose focus.

So hear other people's stories, share in their pain as we are supposed to, but just know that every situation is different. Also know that God has already made provision for your healing by the work He did on the cross. The last words Jesus uttered on the cross were, *"It is finished!"* (John 19:30). Provision has been made for you if you're a Christian. Your sins are forgiven, grace has been supplied, your body is healed, you have access to the peace of God, and the list goes on and on. So since by His stripes you are healed, claim that over your life, along with the other necessary things you must do that require discipline; like changing your eating habits and confessing sins in your life.

I also had to eliminate distractions. I kept myself from people and things that were negative. Just knowing the doctor said I had cancer was bad enough, let alone other things around me that brought my spirit down. The television is just as negative as people can be. It can be hard to remain positive and hopeful when you have the TV on and there's nothing but violence and killing, children being kidnapped, rapes and all sorts of evil. *"And we know that we are of God and the whole world lies under the sway of the wicked one"* (1John 5:19). This world is in such chaos, I had to protect myself from anything that could cause my spirit to be in an uproar. For a short period of time Satan has full range to seek, devour and cause as much disturbance and chaos as he can until his appointed time of destruction in the lake of fire.

What you see and constantly hear has a major affect on where you are in your life, and especially in your mind. To this day I don't watch television much all. When my husband comes home from the office, if he watches a movie, I may watch it with him for the sake of spending time with him. Other than that, I have learned to turn it off or watch something that is inspirational and uplifting. I'm not trying to sound so holy or deep but the fact is, we have control over what we allow in our spirits. Between the spirit and the flesh whichever one you feed the most is the one that grows the most. It's important to keep your spirit fed.

CHAPTER 5

A Life Without Discipline

I read in an article by a guy named Wayne online. He was writing about how advertising creates excess want in a society that doesn't know the meaning of need. As I thought about that, I began to think about commercials and billboards, advertising foods loaded down with grease. Fast foods are loaded with all sorts of harmful preservatives that are dangerous to our bodies. High blood pressure, diabetes, and cancer seem to be on the rise. Commercials and advertising only make the problem worse. We are living in society without discipline.

To put it frankly it not just the commercials. It's the people who have no knowledge of the tricks of the enemy, so when the bad things are being promoted, we think bad is good. Actually, the bad that looks good is causing so much disease and death. The excess want comes from people who have no need, but because they see it, they have to have it, whether it's good for them or not. I really believe that we as people sometimes don't realize the harm we cause ourselves. I know I didn't. Until I was diagnosed I ate whatever I wanted and when I wanted it.

I drank plenty of sodas, I didn't eat many fruits or vegetables, I did absolutely no exercise, and I drank very little water. These are all the things the body needs to defend itself against diseases. So please hear me, if you are a person who takes no thought as to what you and your family are eating, you could be causing great harm to yourself and your loved ones. I didn't write this to scare you, but to be honest; I wish someone had told me what I'm telling you. Healthy eating is very important, whether your goal is to lose weight or not.

This battle made me more compassionate and more aware of the pain in the world. It allowed me to understand fear and heartache like you would never believe. Even though I experienced these emotions, I had complete assurance that God was able to do more than my mind could conceive. *"But through it all and the peace of God which surpasses all understandings will guard your hearts and your mind in Christ Jesus"* (Phil .4:7). I remember one incident when I was resting in the peace of God and the enemy kept making me think that something was wrong with me for not worrying. I was at home with no worries or fear at that time, and sure enough here comes the enemy placing thoughts into my head like; *"you know you should be worrying, because cancer is a deadly disease that many people die from!"*

Instead of casting those thoughts and feelings down; I made a call to my friend Roxanne to ask her if it was it normal for me not to worry about the report the doctors gave. I told her that I felt like I should be worried, and asked if it was normal for me not to worry. These were her exact words; *"You tell that devil that you don't even understand the peace that you have so you know he don't, and that he better back up off you!"* By that time I was pumped up. I said, *"Yea, that's right devil, I don't even understand this peace that I have, so I know you don't. You better back up off me!"*

I got so tickled at her words, but they were so true, and sure enough, those words put the devil under my feet. When the devil tries to play on you and make you think one thing, quickly cast it down. Don't do like I did at that time, listen to him and then question if having peace was possible. The Word of God tells us

"He will keep us in perfect peace whose mind is stayed on Thee" (Isa. 26:3).

This was a tactic of the enemy to keep me fearful, but thank God in my moment of weakness I had a friend close by to encourage me. I was told on numerous occasions that loved ones had found spots on the lungs, cancer on the brain, and every other place that cancer could dwell. I had to continue to trust God even though my expectation didn't match my situation. It became a struggle for me at times to believe God no matter what. God was on the scene but so was the enemy. I was literally fighting the good fight of faith. At moments I found myself to be very strong and then there were times, I felt defeated.

CHAPTER 6

A Call From My Aunt

I received a phone call early one Saturday morning from my aunt Shelia who asked me to read Ezekiel 47:12. I immediately opened my Bible and the Scripture read, *"Along the bank of the river, on this side and that, will grow all kinds of trees used for food; their leaves will not wither, and their fruit will not fail. They will bear fruit every month because their water flows from the sanctuary. Their fruit will be for food and their leaves for medicine."* That scripture gave me fuel to keep going. I had never read it before and was so grateful that she called and asked me to read it. I was so excited and immediately started to praise God, because that Scripture lined up with what I was already doing; which was to eat the food of the earth, and allow it to heal me.

My faith was elevated even more, because now I had a Scripture to back up what I was doing. I had been defiling my temple for years. So many times we think that defilement only comes when we have sex outside of marriage or drinking, but putting the wrong foods in our body is defilement as well. We wonder why there's so much sickness in the earth. Before we start to blame doctors or others; we need to examine ourselves, and take a good look at the things we are taking in.

The next day my family and friends got together for prayer; my aunt anointed and laid hands on me. My brother led us in prayer. The presence of God filled the room, and His spirit assured me that all was well. I kept reminding myself of the Scripture, *"For I know the thoughts that I have for you, says the Lord, plans to prosper you, to give you a future and a hope"* (Jer. 29:11). I had to believe that God was not going to allow this sickness to be the end of me, and that His ultimate master plan would come forth to bring about His glory.

Words that Really Hurt

As I spoke to one of my family members on the phone his first question was, *"You're not dead yet?"* I can't describe to you the pain I felt when I heard those words. Maybe those words were said jokingly, but to me this was definitely no joking matter. We must be careful not to add to a person's pain. If you've never experienced something, and can't sympathize, just say, *"Continue to trust God, or hold on to His promise."* We must be ready at all times for God to use us, even if it's giving a word of encouragement. I was given an apology for the mean words that were spoken, and of course I accepted ,but the words still left its stain. I was the only person in the family who had ever been diagnosed with cancer. I can say this was a learning experience for all of us.

All I could do to keep my mind together was pray and trust God. I found God to be a refuge in the time of trouble. These are not just words, but when things got the hardest for me, I chose to meditate on His Word and found a place of safety. This is a place that you have to get to on your own. Think on His goodness and allow the presence and peace of God to fill your heart and your mind.

Finally, time come for me to have the scans done. I had to sit in this room and drink a white liquid every thirty minutes. The purpose of the liquid was to get a clear look at my colon to see if there was any cancer in that area. The nurse also injected me with sugar water and this would allow them to see where the cancer was in my body. Remember, sugar makes cancer surface so that's why it's very important to reframe from it. After about an hour, I transition to the next room to have the scans done. Everything went well with the scans; now all I had to do was wait for the results. While leaving the doctor's office I met the most beautiful woman with the sweetest spirit I had ever met.

This woman was full of joy and hope. She started telling me about Noah's ark, and how God had dealt with her about being in the ark. She said the ark represented safety. She said God assured her that she was in His care and He was going to bring her through. When she spoke, I listened. She had been through a lot. She had been battling breast cancer for two years. She had no hair, due to the chemo, and had on a matching scarf and hat set. It was evident she was a very classy lady by the way she carried herself. She didn't look or act sick; I could tell that the Lord was with her.

It did my heart good to see her spirits so lifted, and her so encouraged. She had a winning mindset and thus it showed in her attitude. Your mindset is going to be your greatest challenge to overcome and defeat anything in this life. *"As a man thinks in his heart so is he"* (Prov. 23:7). Yes, its true cancer kills hundreds of thousands of people each year, but there is hope, it doesn't matter what type of cancer or what stage it's in. Knowledge is power. The more knowledgeable I became about this disease, the more I knew I could overcome it. Jesus said, *"He has come that we may have life and have it more abundantly"* (John. 10:10). We are not supposed to be defeated in any area of our lives. Sickness, poverty, failure, struggles, no matter what the situation may be; we are supposed to experience the abundant life even in our trials.

CHAPTER 7

My PET and CT Scans

"But with God all things are possible" (Matt. 19:26). As I waited over the next week, I continued to pray and thank God for my healing. I started doing confessions and declaring, *"I will live and not die and declare the works of the Lord"* (Ps. 118:17). I had to keep my thoughts high and was told to keep my future before me. I was determined that my husband and I would do all the things we had planned to do. I would constantly remind myself of God's Word during those moments of fear and doubt as I had to wait patiently for the results.

Lies and Delusions of the Enemy

The devil was busy. I would lie in bed at night and have pains moving throughout my body. The pains would literally be in my elbows, back, and knees. The enemy tried to make me think the cancer was spreading. I told myself I wasn't going to focus on the pain. My focal point was Jesus and the suffering He faced. In spite of how He felt the cross was something He had to face, but with great purpose behind His pain. For the first time in the Bible I saw Jesus at his lowest point. He exemplified strength and power everywhere He went, but in the garden we read about His agony, and His plea for God to let this cup pass from Him.

That gave me comfort to know that it was okay for me to feel agony and dread, as long as my faith was stronger than the fear. As I went back to the doctor for them to give me the results of the recent scans, the cancer was still there, even though I prayed that God would remove it. The cancer was not only there, but it showed another spot on my left leg as well. Yet still the oncologist saw no need to be concerned about the other spot. Praise God, We caught it early and it was in stage one; even with the other spot showing up. I was thanking God that it hadn't spread all over my body.

Better to Trust in God

The oncologists setup another appointment at the cancer center in Greenville. There we met Dr. Matthews, she told us she was concerned about the spot on the other leg, and said that a spot can't just jump from one leg to another leg but that it had to travel. She stated it traveled through my lymph system up my stomach and back down into my leg. And that the cancer was not stage one as earlier diagnosed, but stage two. She suggested chemotherapy as well as radiation; which was completely different from what the previous doctor had said. We were definitely at a cross roads and weren't sure which direction to take. After careful consideration I continued doing what I was already doing.

I told God that I was putting all my faith and trust in Him, and that I didn't want Him to allow anything to happen to me that He didn't ordain. I put my life in the Lord's hands, because I knew He was my healer. I would respect the doctors for their position, but I chose to trust in God. As time went on, I started to do more research on chemo. My mother and my husband had great concerns and weren't in agreement with me taking treatments. I had previously ordered this DVD by Dr. Lorraine

Day; called, *"Cancer, You Don't Scare Me."* She began to expose the hidden side effects of Chemotherapy and Radiation.

Her DVD gave me so much more insight about the damage it causes to the body. She listed so many side effects the oncologist never mentioned. The oncologist basically told us that chemo would make all my hair come out, and that it would cause severe nausea, and I would become very weak. My husband started asking questions like, *"What about chemo destroying the good organs like the heart, liver, and lungs?"* The doctors couldn't deny that it does destroy those organs and couldn't give us any guarantee that those organs would rebuild themselves or that the cancer wouldn't come back.

I thought to myself, *"If there is no guarantee, then why would I put my life at risk and take that chance?"* We found out that chemo causes congestive heart failure, severe kidney damage, sores in the mouth, shortness of breath, pneumonia, memory loss, and so many other serious side effects that the doctors never mentioned. I pray if you or someone you know is faced with the choice to do chemo, that you would do your research. Please don't think that the oncologist has your best interest at heart; some do but most don't. It's his or her job to offer the standard treatment of radiation, chemo, and surgery.

It's not that oncologists aren't sincere in their work. I'm assuming it's the way they've been taught. They aren't allowed to even discuss natural medicines. I spoke with several doctors concerning natural and alternative treatments and was given no comment.

One Friday morning there was a truck explosion on interstate 85; my husband was coming from home to meet me at my appointment by 10:00 a.m. I was already in Spartanburg because I had gotten off from work that morning from third shift. I had been given several diagnoses and now the oncologist wanted to schedule surgery to have the port placed in me.

Since my husband was stuck in traffic I went on the appointment without him. This would be the first time my husband missed any of my appointments. But praise God for my mother who was able to go in his place. She came by my job early that morning and expressed to me that she wasn't feeling comfortable with me taking chemo. She was concerned about the serious side effects and advised me that I shouldn't take it.

By this time I was getting tired. If my mother had not been with me, I was planning on giving in to the treatments; even though I shared the same concerns as her and my husband. For a brief moment I got weary, and it seemed easier to give up than it did to fight. In times like those that's when you need someone who is able to stand up and fight for you if need be.

When we got there, the oncologist expressed his concerns about the treatments. I was strongly urged to take chemo along with radiation, and he said I shouldn't gamble with my life. He then began to make arrangements for me to have surgery and have a port placed into my chest to begin the treatments. My mother immediately said, *"Hold up, I think we need another opinion before we decide to do anything concerning placing ports in her"*. As we left the doctor's office, the staff set us up an appointment at Emory University in Atlanta, Georgia to have another opinion. We found out Emory has an oncologist there who specialized in Hodgkin's, because the oncologist we were seeing specialized in Breast Cancer.

Took My Eyes off God

In the meantime, as I waited for Emory to call me back I would bury myself in God's word. I thought to myself, am *I really going to be able to live day to day knowing this disease is in my body and trust God and act as if it's not?* It's easy to talk about how much we love and trust God, but when our back is against the wall, God is watching to see how our faith holds up. I would have never guessed in a million years that my life would have gone into this direction. God has given to each of us a measure of faith, but this was going to take radical faith. I had to live everyday as if I was already healed until God made it manifest.

My faith was on trial, and I had a lot of people watching me. I spent a lot of time in prayer daily, and His Word gave me strength and comfort that I could not have found in any person. For the most part, I had a very positive outlook on the whole thing. I never looked at myself as being sick. The Scripture is proven *"The spirit of a man will sustain him in sickness"* (Prov. 18:14). God sustained me so much that I never looked sick, I never physically got sick, and even when I had the surgery I never experienced any pain. My greatest challenge was in my mind.

CHAPTER 8

Concealed Information

There is always more than beneath the eye. I learned that even though someone tells you something it seems there is always something being held back. Not one time did the doctor tell me to change my diet or even ask about my diet. They never even mentioned anything about exercise or drinking plenty of water and telling me to cut out all sugar. Surly they had to have known. Everything I found out, I found out on my own. God placed people in my path to let me know what I was doing wrong, or what I should be doing to help myself get well. I continued on in search of anything that I could do to get better, and then trust in due time, all would be well.

In Total Awe

I went to the American Cancer Society for one of their support groups. It was nice to be around other people who were dealing with the same thing. The leader expressed to me how glad she was to have me there. Everyone was very friendly, and I enjoyed meeting and listening to them all. As we continued on, the leader asked me *"Would you like some refreshments while we wait for the rest of the people to get here?"* I said *"sure"* so I went to look and see what type of refreshments there were. I couldn't believe my eyes. There were chocolate chip cookies, brownies and sodas.

I thought to myself *"Why in the world would they serve these types of junk foods to people with this type of illness?"* I thought to myself, *"These people are trying to kill me and everyone else in this room."* Since it was the cancer society, I felt they should have known better than to serve that. Carrots, celery sticks, or even fruit would have been healthier than what they were serving. Everyone there had taken chemo and was in remission and none of them had any idea as to what harm they were causing themselves.

They asked me had I taken chemo or radiation. I told them I had just had surgery to remove the lymph node in March, and I had not taken any treatments. Ms. Laura looked at me and said, *"It seems like you have a long way to go."* I remember looking at her and saying, *"I really don't believe that chemo is the route God wants me to take."* I told them how I had changed my diet and began to look into alternative medicine. Everything I was saying was foreign to them. No one had ever talked to them about anything other than chemo and radiation.

My heart was so heavy because it seemed that none of the doctors had our best interest at heart. I think about so many people who have lost their lives and didn't have to, because the doctors told them like they told me, *"I strongly urge you to take chemo."* I really thought in the beginning that chemo was my only option. So many people to this day still think that. I began to ask people if they knew of anyone who had taken chemo. Everyone knew someone who had taken it, and was either suffering from some other type of illness because of chemo, or who went through it and still died.

If you're reading this book right now, either you have been diagnosed with cancer, or you know someone who was diagnosed. I'm here to tell you there are so many options and chemo is not the only answer. Pray before you think or even react. God will lead you. I'm not telling you not to listen to the doctors, because I feel they are to be respected for their position. I'm just saying there are other options. Don't just take the doctor's word. Talk to the one who created you. He knows your frame inside and out. He will guide you just as He did me. If you have faith to believe all things are possible.

What Does God Say about Healing?

My life had drastically changed. I would get on the internet and look up everything I could about natural healings. I looked up info on Hodgkin's disease and everything associated with it. I looked up herbs, plants, juices, body cleansing and so many other things that would assist me the healing process. All I could think about was how God says, *"My people perish for a lack of knowledge"* (Hosea 4:6). I had to get over the fact that it may have been something that I did wrong to bring about the illness. I chose not to have a pity party, but to keep fighting and keep believing that God was going to heal me. *"But do you want to know, O foolish man, Faith without works is dead"* (James 2:20). I urge you, if you're dealing with cancer; please get up if you can. Do your part by researching, and changing the way you think about cancer. Speak life and encourage yourself. If you can read this book that means you still have breath in your body. It's not over until God says so. This is your chance to take up your bed and walk.

I continued on in my confessions daily: *"I will live and not die and declare the works of the Lord. Lord. You bore my sickness on the cross so that I don't have to bear them. I am whole, complete, and healed by the power of Your word. Your word has given me life. I bind every trace of cancer in the name of Jesus. Every organ, cyst, lymph node, and tissue is healed, and I receive divine healing in Jesus name."* I repeated this confession over and over, and I believed that by the power of my words and thoughts God was going to deliver me from this affliction.

The time I didn't spend reading I spent in the kitchen, juicing, mixing raw vegetables together, and taking natural supplements and herbs around the clock. I would have homemade fruit juice in the morning and a couple of vegetable drinks throughout the rest of the day. I listened to tapes and movies of people who were diagnosed with cancer, and the one thing we didn't have in common was; they would claim the cancer as theirs. I would often hear people say, *"My cancer came back."* *"You are snared by the words of your own mouth"* (Proverbs 6:2) Have you ever wondered why you can't seem to get well? You could be your biggest problem. I urge you to please watch the words that you speak, because it could be those very words that are keeping you bound to sickness. God's Word became my daily bread. Job said, *"I have treasured the words of His mouth more than my necessary food"* (Job. 23:12). I continued my obsession with searching God's word. I started reading about the woman with the issue of blood, and one of the things I realized about her was; she had Jesus on her mind. Jesus was going about as normal healing and performing miracles, but this woman said within herself, *"If I could but touch the hem of His garments, I will be made whole."*

She made her way to Jesus after seeking out doctors and spending all the money she had. She didn't get better, but the Bible says she grew worse. Her story would be a lot different if she had just turned to Him first. She wasted a lot of years and money seeking out her deliverance, when what she really needed was a touch from God. Nonetheless, she heard that Jesus was in town, and made her way to Him. She was very persistent and didn't care who saw her. She was so focused; I can hear her now saying within herself, *"I have nothing else to lose. I've got to get to Him. Lord I'm so tired. I don't care who sees me, I'm so broken Lord, I got to get to You, Lord heal me, Lord heal me!"*

She finally made her way to Him, after pressing her way through the crowd; at last she touched Him! The Bible says the virtue left His body and instantly she was made whole and the flow of her blood dried up (Mark. 5:25-35). Her deliverance was in her pressing. No matter what it is you're going through you must continue to press, and it's during your pressing forth that your faith becomes activated. Notice this woman was on the move; she didn't just lay in her sickness and hope for a miracle. You never know how close you are to your blessing. So labor, labor long if you have to. Be willing to do whatever it takes for however long it takes until your breakthrough comes.

"But without faith it is impossible to please Him, for he who comes to God must believe that He is, and that He is a rewarded of those that diligently seek Him." (Heb. 11:6). This woman believed that Jesus was able to heal her. God has already established who He is. He says I AM whatever you need Me to be. He already is that and more. It's imperative when you receive a bad report from anyone to always turn to God first, because in Him lies your direction, guidance and everything else you will need.

Doctors Sometimes Don't Really Know

Think about it; why should we trust a doctor just because they wear a white coat, and has MD behind their name. When in reality they are complete strangers. We take their word for everything. We let them inject us with needles, and substances that we have no knowledge about. Could it be that we have more faith in the doctors than we have in God our healer? I'm not saying not to take any medicine the doctor gives you. I do believe some medication is needed at times. I'm just saying everything doesn't require medication. Something's require a little more exercise or maybe even changing your eating habits. I really believe that most of the medicine they give us doesn't cure us. It seems it only pacifies the problem. My husband has been on blood pressure medicine for years and he still has blood pressure problems. The medicine hasn't cured him at all.

You would think that since he has been taking two pills everyday for three years or so that he would be high blood pressure-free by now. I'm just saying medicine doesn't really cure. It only curves the symptoms of the sickness. I'm only speaking from my own opinion, but if you think about it, you will see some of the same truths in your own life with people you know or maybe even yourself. *"It's better to trust in God than put confidence in man"* (Ps. 118:8). God has already given us everything we need to heal our- selves with the things of the earth.

We must not be so quick to allow the doctors to prescribe so much medicine especially for our children. The medicine can become addictive and have so many other side effects that can prove to be deadly. We must be swift to pray over ourselves and our children because only God knows what's best for us.

I mean no disrespect to anyone in the health care field, but I've just learned that God is my Physician. It's very important that you shift mentally and understand that everything starts and ends with God. Not with man, so man doesn't have all the answers. To overcome and reverse any illness such as this, it takes the power of God to deliver you, and faith that is a flowing brook. That means your faith has to go beyond where you are, and you must not doubt that nothing is too hard for God. The leper was sure Jesus was more than capable of healing him, but he wasn't sure if it was His will. He asked Jesus, *"Lord if You are willing You can make me clean, and Jesus, moved with compassion, put forth His hand and touched him, and said unto him, I am willing, be thou clean"* (Mark. 1:40, 41).

The promises of God says, *"above all, I wish that thou mayest prosper and be in good health even as thy soul prospers"* (3 John 1:2). This Scripture, along with plenty others clearly states that God intends for us to have good health and prosperity. Sickness is demonic. It's of the devil and we don't have to accept it into our lives. On the other hand, sometimes God does allow sickness when we are living in direct violation of the will of God, and sickness is used sometimes as a tool to get us to repent and put us back in right relationship with God.

"*If you diligently heed the voice of the Lord your God, and do what is right in His sight, give ear to His commandments and keep all His statues, I will put none of the diseases on you which I have brought on the Egyptians; for I am the Lord who heals you*"(Exod. 15:26). I have come to learn that we are not our own; we have been brought at a high price. We belong to God, and that means obeying His commandments and statues. Otherwise the consequences can be detrimental. So right now, if you are sick or going through anything major in your life, examine yourself as well as the situation.

CHAPTER 9

The Purpose of Suffering

The footnotes in the Open New King James Study Bible say; God allows sufferings for different reasons. Sometimes it's a situation like Job, which is to prove to the enemy you will serve God now matter what. Other times it could be a situation we have brought on ourselves. At times we don't know what's in us until we experience suffering. I always thought that my passion was working with teenage girls, which I still love, but a new passion has been birth in me.

I am more passionate about educating people about this intruder called cancer. Way too many people are dying because they trusted the doctors instead of God. We as people need to become more educated on the foods we allow to enter our bodies that are causing us a slow death that will manifest down the line. God's purpose for our lives has already been established before the foundations of the world. What you're going through right now may have caught you off guard, but there are no surprises with God. Even if it's something we have caused ourselves, our God is still faithful and stands ready to deliver us.

I felt that I was bound by this sickness. As I choose to trust God, I knew that it was a process I would have to go through.

All I could think at times was, *I want this cancer out of me!* I would have my moments where I became distant, followed by a stream of tears. I had a few moments when I took my eyes off of God and began to focus on the cancer; then I became extremely fearful. After all, a lot of people had died from this disease; and the enemy tried to make me think I was next. *"God had not given me the spirit of fear but of power, love and a sound mind"* (2Tim. 1:7).

The enemy wasn't letting up, but in the midst, God gave me a revelation: *"He that is in you is greater than he that is in the world"* (1John 4:4). I realized that since the greatness of God dwells in me, and God is all-powerful, then the power of God and sickness can't reside in the same temple. The power of God would rise up in me, and I would put the devil under my feet where he belonged. My Aunt Shelia kept telling me to stand on God's Word no matter what, and to know I was healed.

I would continue to bind Satan and his demons and loose God's healing power in my life. *"Whatever you bind on earth will be bound in heaven and whatever you loose on earth will be loosed in heaven"* (Matt. 6:19). I was willing to do whatever it took to get well. I knew that *death and life are in the power of the tongue (Proverbs 18:23),* and that we have the power to create our world, just as God did in the beginning. I had to open my mouth and continue to declare my healing. I decided that I wanted my world to be full of good health and prosperity, just as God desires for us. So I had to bind my own thoughts at times, and well any negative vibes I got from anyone else. I really had to spend time loosing God's protection over me, and asking Him to cover me in His blood. I felt extremely safe under the blood. Please I urge you, if you can, cover yourself always. Constantly plead the blood of Jesus over your life because there are demonic forces working in the unseen realm of the spirit that are sent and assigned to destroy you.

The Process of Examination

It didn't take me long to realize what causes cancer. Through my research, I found that a diet high in fat, saturated fats, sugar, lack of nutrients in the body, lack of fruits and vegetable, lack of exercise, stress, smoking, lack of water, genetics, chemicals, metal, radiations, and pesticides in our food; are all contributing factors as to what causes cancer. I also started seeing a woman named Terry. She owns her own store in downtown Greenville and specializes in Natural foods, and holistic medicines. She began to guide me and show me other things that I could take and do to get rid of the cancer. This woman was truly God sent. God used her not only to help me through cancer. He used her to help me with the emotions that followed. She literally became my nutritionist/counselor/friend. In fact this book is dedicated to her.

If you or a loved has been diagnosed with cancer, I think you owe it to yourself, and to them to find out as much information about this disease as possible. So many people to this day are still ignorant as to what causes cancer. Now of course we don't know everything, but whatever the situation is, do your own research. The more knowledgeable you are about it, the more confident you will feel that you can overcome it. No matter what the doctor's tell you, I guarantee there will be things they won't tell you. The Internet and books are a great source for researching.

We can't just blame the doctors, because we are the ones who take their word. No matter what type of cancer it is, their method of treatment is all the same. There are different drugs for different types of cancer, but none of them guarantee you're healing. It's like playing rushing roulette with your life. I understand that some things aren't certain, but the treatments that the oncologist offers have way too many side effects. It's just too risky. It seems there have been more people who have died from the treatments, than there is who has lived because of them.

Three months is all it should take to turn any situation around, concerning your health. This will require discipline, and a complete life style change. I went to a seminar for Natures Sunshine in Asheville NC. I sat through a class as our digestive system was being discussed. There I found out herbs change the environment of the body so that it can begin to heal itself. If we stop feeding our body the bad foods, the disease will leave. Rats won't live in a clean home. Another thing that plays a huge part in sickness is our emotions.

There are only two basic emotions that we all experience, love and fear; all other emotions variations of these two emotions. Thoughts and behavior come from either a place of love or a place of fear. Anxiety, anger, control, sadness, depression, inadequacy, confusion, hurt, loneliness, guilt, shame, all of these are fear based emotions. Emotions such as, joy, happiness, caring, trust, compassion, truth, contentment and satisfactions, these are all love based emotions.

When you are experiencing fear, it damages the immune system, the endocrine system and every other system in our bodies. Our immune system becomes weaken and many serious illnesses set it. When you are in love your body releases special chemicals that make you feel strong, content, happy and able to conquer the world.

Each day we take in about 20,000 breaths and about thirty pounds of air. A single sneeze can send more than five thousand respiratory droplets into the air, at a speed of forty seven. We are taking in so much from the environment we live in. It is very important to keep your body well hydrated with plenty of water. We must concentrate on deep slow breaths, and do everything we can to alleviate stress.

God says *"My people perish for a lack of knowledge."* (Hosea 4:6). There has always been a saying, *"What you don't know can't hurt you"* We'll I'm here to tell you, what you don't know can hurt you, and even kill you. Fran Drescher, as she battled uterine cancer wrote something in her book Cancer Schmancer; that was an eye opener for me: *"We are the ones who must change, if we expect there to be change."* We must take control of the situation and become educated people. Know your body, if there is a knot or some type of tenderness you have noticed, get it checked out. Let's not assume, and certainly not say within yourself *"oh it's nothing."* The very thing that you think could be nothing, could turn out to be something life threatening.

My body was full of all the wrong things, and not to be too gross, but I was having a very hard time with regular BMs. This is also another contributing factor. As food goes in, it must come out. This is the process of elimination. Hodgkin's disease is a disease in the body that affects the lymphatic system; which is a part of the body's immune system that helps the body fight off disease and infection. The two avenues that cancer enters the body are through the fluid systems, which involve the lymphatic system and the blood system.

No one is exempt from cancer. As a matter of fact, we all have cancer cells growing in our bodies every day but not everyone will develop cancer. One of the differences between someone who has cancer and someone who doesn't is the immune system wasn't able to fight off the disease and therefore cancer developed. That's why I began to take a lot of supplements and eat food that targeted my immune system. I knew that if I could get that built back up, along with eating right and making sure I remained in a healthy emotional state. I had a good chance of reversing the cancer. It wasn't hard, and in fact, I believe it kept me from showing the symptoms from the cancer.

I started looking over a list of the chemotherapy drugs the oncologist gave me, and for every drug there was a long list of side effects. This puzzled me because how could a medicine that is supposed to make you get well have so many dangerous side effects? I also was given a book called Eating Hints for Cancer Patients, and it talked about complementary medicines, which are natural herbs and supplements. It says the medicine given for cancer has not been proven safe, and if one spent time taking complementary medicines, one may lose valuable treatment time and reduce one's chances of controlling the cancer and getting well. Based upon my research, I haven't read any stories where natural medicines have caused serious life threatening side effects.

The oncologist may put pressure on you and make you think that time is wasting and you must go ahead with the traditional treatments. They told me not to gamble with my life, and strongly urged me to take chemo. Praise God, I waited about three weeks before I made any decision. I didn't care what they thought or said. During that time, I prayed and allowed God to lead me. I'm so thankful that I had a mind not to fret, but chose to turn to God. I perceived that God was my healer and I refuse to let go of Him until my healing came forth. I couldn't imagine my healing coming from something that could make me worse off than I already was.

How can something that supposed to make you well turn out to be so deadly? Why is it legal for the doctor's to administer it? The surgeon never educated me on the infection in my body, which later turned out to be Hodgkin's Disease/cancer. All he said was there was an infection, and it was in my lymph nodes, and they weren't certain of the cause right then.

God's Medicine

"And God said, See I have given you every herb that yields seed which is on the face of all the earth, and every tree whose fruit yields seeds: to you it shall be for food" (Gen 1:29). Even though there are so many different causes and types of cancer, I believe all of it could have been prevented with the proper diet. God has given us our food, and in our food are all the nutrients the body needs to maintain good health. Think about it, when a dog is sick, he begins to eat grass. When humans get sick, why do we turn to chicken noodle

soup, and immediately run to physicians? We should turn to the foods of the earth; such as leafy greens and vegetables, as well as fruit. We should also be taking some form of multivitamin as a precautious measure.

When Adam and Eve were in the Garden of Eden their food consists of the food of the earth. "He causes the grass to grow for the cattle, and vegetation for the service of man, that he may bring forth food from the earth." *(Ps.* 104: 14). Everything that God created He called good. There is nothing polluted about it, at least not then. It's not even safe to go to the grocery store and buy anything off the shelves. I know this is a shock to you. I especially want to talk with the mothers, because they are the ones grocery shopping and bringing the food home and cooking for the entire family.

Women are feeding processed foods and meats loaded with hormones and chemicals in them to their families. This could be taken as a harsh statement, but this is only my opinion. I really feel that, because of the foods that women buy and cook for their families, they could be killing their families and not even realizing it. An environment in our bodies is being created that disease can run rapid in. Remember God says *"My people perish for a lack of knowledge."* Parents, spend some extra time in the grocery stores reading the ingredients of the foods you purchase. You will learn more at the end of the book about certain ingredients to watch out for.

CHAPTER 10

According to Your Faith

A woman spoke so profoundly when she said; *"Different paths are laid out for different people and sometimes it through no fault of our own."* Whatever the cross you may be carrying; it was designed for you, and you had no choice in the matter." Now I realize that this present situation was pre-sent before the foundations of the world. God knew exactly what my struggles and trials were going to be. He also knew how I would react while going through, and He knows the same for you. There are some something's we can't avoid, especially if it's going to be used for other people's deliverance and bring about His glory.

This was my cross that I had no choice but to carry. Only God knows your beginning and your ending. He knows the pain and suffering that we will have to endure. Whatever the situation maybe, God is on the throne and has ultimate control of our lives. So be not afraid, because we overcome our fears and our trials by our faith in God and His word.

You may be thinking, now what does that mean? That means, we don't have to be afraid of anything that comes our way. The Bible is full of promises that were made to them that would believe them. Just as the law was written for law breakers, the promises of God are written to them that would believe them. If God has made provision for your healing on the cross; why would you accept sickness?

Everything you desire; whether it be good health, bills paid, peace of mind, promotion on your job, husband or wife saved; whatever the situation maybe; let it be unto you according to your faith. Faith and fear can't operate in the same situation. Either you are fearful or you will have faith enough to believe. Fear causes too much torment; faith causes you to have peace. If you find yourself always worried and reasoning within yourself, then it's a good chance you have let fear get the best of you. Doubt and fear is a sneaky thing because so many people operate in it and don't realize it. Their up at night, walking the floors, stressed out, depressed, and feeling defeated and most of the time you won't realize these emotions, until you have gotten sick, or someone tells you.

I had the privilege of being used by God to minister to other women and men who were battling cancer. I had come to believe if God led me to a person who was sick, that He wanted to heal them. I talked with countless people who had already adopted a defeated mindset. Most of them had cancer years before and the cancer had returned. I begin to speak about faith in God, and trusting in Him for their healing. I spoke of natural supplements and diet change but what amazed me was; how just about everyone hung onto the doctors reports. Who will stand up and believe the report of the Lord? It's not my job to persuade or influence anyone to do as I did. I can only share my faith.

I heard Dr. Mike Murdock say something that was so profound. He said, *"It's our faith that decides God's divine timing in our life."* That really ministered to me because so many times we say it's all in God's time, and I do believe that everything is according to His divine timing. It's also means the sooner you act in faith and believe God for your miracle, the sooner your miracle comes forth.

There is a Methodist church down the street from my home. I have noticed at least once a month there is a sign posted out front that says, *"Healing service tonight 7:00 p.m."* This one day in particular, around 6:15 that evening; I rode past and saw the sign. I immediately told myself that I was going, and had forty five minutes to get myself together and get back to the service by seven. When I got home, I had quickly talked myself out of it. While I was in the kitchen, this pain went through my stomach and I fell to the floor, *"Okay Lord, I hear You"* I said to myself. I hurried up and got my things together and left the house. When I got there I was the only black person in the church, and everyone was much older than I was.

I had never been to a church like this before, but I also never felt the love God like I had experienced Him there. We sang songs, did communion, there were prayer requests being offered up, and they asked everyone to come to the altar, and kneel in prayer. What really touched me was; they had all the elders at the front of the church and asked anyone if they would like to come up front and have the elders pray with them. I went up front. There were two women and one man standing with me. One lady immediately asked me, *"What is your favorite color"* I told her *"green"*. There was a lady in the back of the church making quilted blankets. I picked out a green blanket and the elders wrapped me up in this blanket as they stood around me.

They said to me, *"Anytime you feel afraid, or need to feel the presence and the peace of God, wrap yourself in this blanket."* They asked me what I needed prayer for. I told them that *"the doctors told me I had cancer, and I believe God to heal me without chemo and radiation."* They stood in agreement with me and began to pray one by one for me. As I stood there in the middle of them, I could only cry as I felt the presence of the Lord in me and surround me. The prayers were so sweet and the people were so genuine. That experience was one that I will never forget. I left there very encouraged as I continued to stop at nothing to obtain divine health.

I heard Apostle Ron Carpenter speak about Representation. He said if God was going to do anything in the earth, He would work through people. Why is it the people of God aren't laying hands on the sick just as the Bible tells us to? Why aren't there more services just about healing? I realized this was much needed. Could it be that we don't have the faith to believe that God can work through us. I thought at one point just because my healing hadn't manifested yet I couldn't lay hands on anyone, but I was so wrong. It seemed that God really begin to use me during that time.

In the name of Jesus

There is power In the name of Jesus. If you haven't tried using His name, try it. Use it with faith and assurance. Declare and decree that cancer has to bow down. You may have to say it over and over at times. Do this along with the other things that are suggested to bring forth your healing. God told Moses to use what he had in his hand. Moses had everything he needed to perform the task at hand; we to have everything that we need. We just have to realize that we already have it.

For all us it will take opening up our mouth, claiming victory in the middle the situation. You are literally going to battle with the forces from the unseen. You have to know that you have the victory before you go, and understand that the battle is not yours but the Lords. So be encouraged and take your stand. Take back what the enemy is trying to steal from you. No matter what the situation maybe, you are victorious!

CHAPTER 11

My Spiritual Weapons

You must get God's word in your spirit and use it as your weapon against the enemy. Your mouth is a weapon because *"life and death are in the power of the tongue"* (Prov.18:21). You can have what you declare if you believe you have already received it by faith. You receive it by believing the promises of God. When Jesus cursed the fig tree, the leaves didn't wither away right then. He spoke the words, and later what He spoke began to manifest. I said that to say you may be declaring God's Word and speaking it over and over, and just because your healing hasn't manifested, don't stop declaring and please don't stop believing that you have your healing.

It's done. You must continue to wait on the manifestation of it, and remember consider not how you may be feeling. God's Word is true. If He said it, then it is so! *"Heaven and earth will pass away but, My word will stand forever"* (Isa. 40:8). After all, we are talking about cancer here. I've heard of people calling cancer the "big C", but I know a man who is able to make even cancer bow down. His name is Christ, and He's the real "big C". In fact God is so mighty you can't drown Him, because He will just walk on water. You can burn Him up, because He will take the flame out of the fire. There is nothing that He can't do, He's an awesome all Powerful God!

How do you see Jesus? Do you perceive Him to be the Son of man or the Son of God? If you perceive Him to be the Son of man then you see Him as being Joseph's son; you believe there is nothing powerful about Him. If you believe Him to be the Son of God, then you know there's nothing too hard for Him, and that He stands ready and able to deliver you.

I chose life

Even though I knew that God was all powerful, and I perceived Him to be my healer. I continued to fight the good fight of faith. I continued on proclaiming my healing but the thorn in my flesh was deep. I was often told that I was a very strong person, but at times I sure didn't feel so strong. My soul was in agony, and I felt the pangs of death all around me. From time to time I would say to myself *"Shell are you crazy, what in the world made you think you could beat this cancer without the recommended chemo and radiation treatments?"* I didn't doubt the decision not to do treatments, because even though the doctor said that it was curable, I had come to believe my healing wasn't coming forth through the standard treatment. I had been doing everything to get well. When I left the Methodist Church, I felt complete assurance, but as time went on the enemy crept back in. At times I was very strong in the Lord and other times I was in despair. After all, I was in the fight of my life.

All I could think about was the Scripture *"The thief cometh to steal, kill and to destroy, but Jesus said I am come that you may have life and have it more abundantly"* (John. 10:10). In my mind chemo was the work of the enemy. It severely destroys the immune system, along with good functioning organs, and for some people it even kills. God can turn any situation around; so if you or a person you know has already begun chemo treatments, there are natural supplements you can take that may keep your immune system built up. It's a possibility the supplements will help fight off the disease, and begin to rid your body of the poisoning from the treatments, and possibly at the same time reverse the cancer. I must say it is definitely harder to treat cancer with natural medicines if chemo has already been used, but God can still turn any situation around.

I decided to go with life more abundantly, so I had to continue standing and trusting in God. I had to stand trusting Him or die believing Him, but chemo and radiation were not an option. My mind at one point began to play tricks on me. In my imagination I saw myself as If I had died, and honestly I entertained the thoughts of suicide at one point. I know these weren't my thoughts-they were of the enemy, and I had to catch myself, and then I had to put Satan under my feet. At times I would take a look at my life, and it was as if I was watching a movie. It just didn't seem real.

One day I went to sleep, and when I woke up my whole world was turned upside down. I looked at the people around me who seemed as if they didn't have a care in the world. People shopping, laughing, my husband going to work as usual; everyone seemed to be going on with their daily activities, but I felt my life had come to a halt. All I could think about was getting well and my actions were geared toward that. I spent hours each day in prayer, loosing God's healing in my life.

I wondered to myself Lord is this end of me? As a matter of fact, when the doctor told me I had cancer, I asked him was I going to die. I cried out *"Lord please no!"* I haven't even been married a year at that time, and my husband and I had so much that we wanted to do. We had a trip to San Diego California planned for August. I was determined I was going, and going cancer free at that, so I had to get a grip and keep fighting.

CHAPTER 12

Just What I Needed

My brother gave me a CD from a revival at a church he had attended. The title of his message was *"No Pain, No Glory."* Just the title alone ministered to me. Basically, if I was going to be used by God, I would have to endure some pain and suffering. I told God if this is the cup that I have to drink, I will drink it. People kept telling me *"God is going to use you to minister to other people in the same situation."* I remember going to my sister's wedding and driving to Florida. On the way back it began to rain cats and dogs. I had gotten to a point while I was driving, I couldn't see the road. I saw people with their blinkers on driving slowly; while others had stopped completely because of the rain.

Even though cancer was my storm, I couldn't stop. I could have pulled over; meaning give up, feel hopeless, defeated and accept the doctor's report, but I chose to put my blinkers on, take it a little bit slower and seek God for direction.

This was the season that I was in. However, I don't believe a Christians life, is one of continual suffering. Some Christians believe that if they aren't suffering, then something must be wrong with their relationship with God. Yes it's true the Bible says *"If we suffer with Him, we will reign with Him"* (2 Tim. 2:12). So there are going to be times of suffering, along with times of peace, and happiness. I went through my season of suffering, but even in the midst of that, I still had a reason to praise God. I encourage you, if you're going through look for reasons to praise God. The enemy of sickness and death can be destroyed because of your praise.

We are all going to leave this earth someday. Yes, Jesus defeated death on the cross, that means; if you are a true Christian, even though our bodies will all one day return to the dust of the earth, our spirit will live on forever, with our Father in Heaven.

I wouldn't trade this experience for the world. God is faithful, if He brings you to it, He will bring you through it. Our life is a journey and we are constantly changing and growing. I encourage you to keep walking, keep praying, and continue believing. You're not going anywhere until God's appointed time. God through Jesus is affiliated with your pain. He knows exactly how you feel, and stands ready to deliver you. It is always my desire to please God, by my acts of faith. *"And he believed in the Lord, and He was accounted it to him for righteousness."*(Gen.15:6). When Abraham was asked to offer his only son Isaac up for sacrifice; God was pleased with his faith. God provided a ram to be offered up instead. It was only a test. What you're going through right now could be a test. Are you passing or failing? Do you believe God is pleased with how you are handling whatever the situation you may be faced with, or do you find yourself complaining?

It wasn't anything that I did so great that God would show me His favor. We can't earn righteousness by our good works. God loves us in spite of what we do, and what we don't do. However, you can please God by having steadfast faith in Him. Think about, what else do you have to lose? Some people are extremely wealthy, but when it comes down to it; our money doesn't earn us any extra rewards. If you're fortunate enough to live a long life, you certainly can't take money with you. Get yourself together, and turn to God. Ask Him to show you how to take care of yourself, and to be mindful of the things that really matter. You only have one body here on earth.

Let's take care of the temple that God has given us by putting the right things in our bodies. I learned that God allowed the pain in my body to remind me, that there has been a diagnosis. If I was going to believe God, my faith had to be tested to see if I would focus on the pain, or trust Him through it all. God remained close because He knew that I chose to trust in Him. Even when things seem the darkest and the hour is late that's when God begins to turn things around.

We serve a God who doesn't sleep or slumber, so why should we lie awake at night worrying about something that ultimately God has control over? I chose victory over defeat, and I knew that my life was in the Master's hand. Victory only comes through battle, and triumph follows trials. To me victory was living through it all and being able to help and see someone else through, and that person can help bring someone else through.

I would be victorious if I came out with a stronger faith than I ever had, and a closer relationship with God and my family. That would be the sweet taste of victory for me. My husband endured like a true solider and stood by me the whole time. I praise God for the awesome man of God that he is. He made sure he went on all my appointments except when he was stuck in traffic. He nurtured and provided not only the tangible things but also the love and support. My sister, mother, and aunt showed compassion and longsuffering like I never expected, praise God!

CHAPTER 13

When I Looked Around

I learned that everyone that starts out with you is not always the ones who will see you through. When I first received the diagnosis I had people who were there praying with me, and believing God with me, but somehow along the way some people became scarce. God has people in our lives for seasons and different reasons. I have to say through this process I have learned to put all my faith in God, because people will let you down, and I really don't believe that anyone intends to. It's just everyone can't see what you see, and everyone can't feel what you feel.

Therefore this can cause people to become distant if they can't relate to what you're going through. I urge you as you read this book, step outside yourself, and learn to labor with people until their break through comes. If you're the one going through it, keep believing God until your break through comes. Go ahead and start thanking God now for your healing. I heard Dr. Mike Murdock say that the reasons why a lot of people don't get the things they ask God for is, because they don't labor long enough until it comes.

They give up too quickly. They feel if God hasn't done it in a certain amount of time, then He's not going to. This causes you to miss out on what you believe God for. We don't get weary but we believe God for the greatest outcome for however long it takes. Even though I went through this, I praise God for all things, because He knows what you need just when you need it. He allowed Oral Roberts Ministry to be there as a strong support system. They would send me information in the mail. I received calls from their prayer partners asking me if I needed them to touch and agree with me about anything that day.

How I stayed encouraged

Pastor Roberts and his wife Lindsey sent me a CD with nothing but Scripture on it. Their instructions were to listen to it over and over until the Word got down on the inside of me. He allowed me to meet up with people of great faith to lay hands on me and anoint me. As I looked back I could see how everything was strategically set up by God. God gave me songs that kept me encouraged. "To be Kept by Jesus" by Juanita Bynum, "Jesus" by Shekinah Glory, "Resting on His Promises" by Youthful Praise, and "All I need" by Brian Courtney Wilson were all the songs that God used to minister to me.

Every time I heard those songs, I grew so much strength and my faith was lifted even higher. The one thing about this faith walk is that your faith will not stay the same. Your faith will be challenged and become elevated. Remember "*faith cometh by hearing and hearing by the word of God*" (Rom. 10:17). The more I heard and read God's Word, the more I believed His word. I began to go online and look up different ministries and listen to different sermons on healing. I even tuned in to Benny Hinn's website as God used Him to lay hands on the sick (Mark 16:18). I could literally feel the anointing, and the power of God through the monitor. I would go to church with expectations, and wait for the Word to come forth.

I allowed the Word of God to minister to me. I became desperate for it, because I knew in it was life. Most of the time I had to research, seek out and study the Word on my own, I was determined that this cancer was getting out of my body. I would anoint myself daily as well as take communion. I wasn't playing. I did every act of faith imaginable to receive my healing. Maybe I left the door open by not eating right, and being under so much stress from the month of December, or maybe God was allowing this for His greater purpose either way God was going to be glorified!

I know that God does not seek to interfere with our happiness, but He does require that we relinquish our will, for He cannot bless us as He desires to do until our will is yielded up, and we accept His in exchange. Jesus gave up His will in the garden of Gethsemane, *"Not my will but Thy will be done."* God has a perfect will for your life. So many times we are in resistance to what God is doing. When we resist the process we're tampering with God's plan. We never know whose deliverance we are holding up, including our own.

It's my job as well as yours to go and strengthen our brother when God brings us through. Look at Jesus on the cross; the way that He suffered and died was through no fault of His own, but the world through Him may have eternal life. The whole world gained because of the things that He suffered.

God used this situation to draw my family closer. My mother and I grew even closer as we often discussed the things that I researched. She loved it when I called her, and shared with her the things I found out during my research on cancer. My aunt believed I was healed when I didn't know that I was healed according to God's Word. She spoke life and encouragement to me constantly. My sister called me every day to see how I was feeling and exemplified so much compassion. So you see so much good came out of my trials, and now praise God my very first book has come out of them.

Back in Winston Salem

The time came for us to be in Winston Salem. It was June by this time. I didn't dread being there, but somehow it did strike up old memories. Like I said earlier, I found the lymph node while in Winston Salem in January. From January to June everything had completely changed. Little did I know at the time I found the knot in my thigh that all this was going to take place. A lot of pain, frustration and healing had taken place within those six months. I thought to myself, *this is where it all began.*

While I was in my room once again my husband was downstairs at the RVP meeting. I began to praise and thank God, because even though I was going through what I was going through, God was bringing me through it, and I dared not complain. I had no other attitude except for gratefulness, because from January until then, I had come through a lot, but at least I was still here. I actually felt better than I had ever felt in my life. The diet change along with exercising was a much needed change. Through exercising I actually found a new way to relax and mentally distress.

I have had women and men ask me if I would help them with weight loss, because I had lost so much weight. I proceeded to tell them to cut out all sugars and breads to start with, and drink only water with plenty exercise on a regular basis. The exact words I get most of the time are, "*You mean to tell me no sweets?*" Once again, our desire gets us in trouble because everything that's good isn't good for you. However, there are people who took my advice and actually began to lose their weight and feel healthier.

I hear people say all the time there aren't enough hours in a day. Unfortunately, there are always going to be things that keep us distracted. This world is so demanding, and we are often pulled into so many directions. We must be willing to change. We can't change the direction we're going in until we change the way we think. This often calls for us to make conscious efforts. Some things are more important than others. I would say our health takes top priority, so we must exercise ourselves in the Lord first by reading and studying His Word on a daily basis. Second exercise and take care of our physical bodies.

I read on the American Cancer Society Website; that over five hundred thousand people die a year of cancer, and thousands of people are being diagnosed with it every day. This disease is aggressively ruining our country. We must stop taking our health for granted and be mindful of what we are putting into our bodies. Get the heads up on the disease now and start taking preventive measures for you and your family. If not there's no guarantee that we will be around to see the rich fulfillment that God has for you. Life offers no guarantees, but the promises of God are sure.

CHAPTER 14

Walking Right Before God

There's nothing that gets God attention more than the suffering of one of His saints. *"Many are the afflictions of the righteous but the Lord delivers us out of them all"* (Ps. 34:19). I have to say there are some steps that we must take when believing God for your healing. First, you must confess any sins you may have, and turn from them. Have no unforgiveness in your heart or any bitterness toward anyone. If you expect to get God's attention you have to come before Him clean; let God see that you want Him not just for what He can give or do for you. I know if I expect Him to move on my behalf I must live according to His Word, but I had to study His Word in order to know how to live by it. How else could I expect God to deliver me if I'm not keeping His word and desiring Him on a daily basis?

God has a perfect will and a plan for our lives and at some point we all will face some suffering. When we suffer for righteousness's sake, God is after something that only suffering can produce, and bring forth. Suffering has a tendency to produce tunnel vision; it produces more fruit, compassion, vision, direction, and so many other things. Be careful not to murmur and complain while you're going through, because that could be the very thing that's keeping you suffering.

I took a look at Job's life. The Bible says that he was a perfect and upright man, one who feared God and shunned evil. Job suffered for no wrongdoings of his own. God allowed Satan to have his way with Job to prove to the enemy that Job wasn't serving Him for material things. Job had his moments where he wondered what was going on; he doubted himself but never God. When we are faced with different trials, we must have the patience and endurance that Job had. Every trial is not sent to destroy you, but sometimes God uses your sufferings to silence the devil.

"Before I was afflicted I went astray but now I keep your word" (Ps. 119:67). Sometimes sufferings are sent by our Heavenly Father as a consequence of our sin. Just as our earthly father must chastise us when we disobey, so does our Father in Heaven. But think about it. God loves us so much that He doesn't immediately destroy us in our sin. He sends warning before destruction every time. *"The Lord is not slack concerning His promise, as some count slackness, but is longsuffering toward us, not willing that any should perish, but that all should come to repentance"* (2 Pet. 3:9). I love this scripture, because it clearly shows His desire for all of His creation to be with Him in paradise. God if He wanted to could immediately destroy us in our sins, but because we were created for Him and by Him, every day that He allows up to wake up, is another opportunity to repent and turn to Him. God is a perfect example of longsuffering.

Suffering can also be sent at times to teach us to lean and depend on God. It's sad to say, but true if we are not suffering with some sort of sickness, financial problem or some kind of heartache we would hardly ever look to God. The fact of the matter is, most people don't accept Christ into their lives until they are down and out, and experiencing hardship. That's why you hear so many stories of men and women getting saved while they're in jail. Although there is nothing wrong with that, God knows what it is going to take to get our attention. We need suffering sometimes to keep us near the cross. When we experience suffering, we pray more, we study God's Word more, and we learn to lean and depend on Him in ways we never did before.

When I was diagnosed with cancer I felt I had been betrayed by my own body. I had experienced people turning on me, but never my own body; after all this was the same body that I had been taking care of since I could take care of myself. At first I thought what am I going to do? I couldn't doubt that God was going to heal me. As my appearance changed, I begin to see myself differently. I think the hardest part of having cancer was losing all the weight, but for most people that would have been the easiest part. I begin to relive my childhood all over again. As a child I was always very thin, and use to get teased a lot about it. It didn't matter if anyone told me I looked good, it was how I saw myself. My husband experienced the pain of not being able to take the cancer from me, and expressed his helplessness as a man wanting to fix it for me.

CHAPTER 15

Bearing Fruit

I had previously watched the movie *Temptations,* and one of the singers mother was diagnosed with cancer. She said; *"she was feeling fine until the doctor's started curing her, and that the treatment was worse than the disease."* You may say that I watch too much TV, but based on my research and talking with cancer patients and their families; it's true the treatment is worse than the disease. I'm not telling you not to take the treatments, but be sure whatever you decide, you have prayed about it, and have peace with whatever you decide.

God said, *"I am the true vine and My Father is the vinedresser. Every branch in Me that does not bear fruit He takes away; and every branch that bears fruit He prunes, that it may bare more fruit"*(John 15: 1, 2). Jesus wasn't talking about fruit that you purchase from a store. He was talking about the fruit that produces righteousness and holiness in God our Father. I realized God was after something in me. He must have been if I am supposed to bear fruit, but I knew I had to stay connected to the Vine. Through tribulations God is bringing His chosen ones into perfection, that we may bear the fruit that is pleasing to the Father, and draw others to Christ. Once again, it's all through the Vine. I urge you get connected and stay connected, *"For in Him we live, move and have our being"* (Acts 17:28).

We must have courage, and trust that God will sustain us. God is our only source. His word says, *"These signs will follow them that believe, they will lay hands on the sick and they shall recover"* (Mark. 16:18). God gave us the power, but it was by faith that we receive it. It's not in the actual physical touch of the hands but the healing comes by the power and the authority of God as we are connected to Him.

A Home Visit

Ministry took hold of me. It was no longer about my pain and suffering. God really began to send me forth to speak and encourage others. This was the ultimate act of faith, and of course the ultimate reward. I couldn't look to my own natural abilities. I was empowered by the Spirit as I continued to walk in faith. I remember going to this woman's home that had breast cancer. Now like I said earlier, I believed if God sent me to a person He wanted to heal them. I got to the home of Ms. Gladys. She was a beautiful lady who had cancer years earlier, but the cancer returned. God used me to minister to her and her family. Her husband was very quiet and also very attentive. I'm sure he was curious as to why I was there. Their daughter Sharon was a good friend of mine. She knew some of the things I had been through and thought I could share my faith and my experience to help her mother.

I could tell her mother and father had never heard of anyone being healed from cancer without the standard medicine. I spoke with the family, and shared my faith. I could see that Ms. Gladys began to be encouraged. She asked me *"how did I get started on the natural path?"* By the time I was getting ready to answer her, a commercial came on television. It was First Lady Reva McCluney, and Pastor promoting a commercial for their church

(New Harvest). I immediately lit up and said; *"That's the lady who shared her faith with me, and when I didn't know what I was going to do, God used her and I received direction!"* That was my first time seeing their commercial, and it confirmed in that moment God was in the midst of everything I was doing.

I continued to talk with the family, and tell them some things they could do and some different teas Ms. Gladys could drink. To make a long story short, upon my leaving I felt the need to lead the family in prayer. As the prayer was being prayed, the power of God filled the room. Ms. Gladys's husband had a whole different demeanor, and by the time I left I could see he was encouraged. He was smiling and felt very hopeful, praise God!

I received a call from my husband telling me a woman named Ms. Jackie had liver cancer. He wanted to know would I be willing to speak with her. *"Of course"* I said, helping people became my focus. I called Ms. Jackie and we scheduled a time to meet. This was a very sweet spirited and quiet spoken woman. She had been to several doctors who showed a lack of compassion during her visits. Anyhow, she was tired and needed help. Once again God used me, I began to explain to her about her diet and things she needed to stop eating. I immediately referred her to Terry; there she received more guidance about reversing the cancer. Within months praise God, Ms. Jackie was cancer free. She took no chemo or radiation. She changed the way she was eating and started taking natural supplements. I give God all the praise and Glory for this.

At times we all will deal with some serious problems, but it's your attitude that will determine your outcome, and how soon you come out of your problem. It's about how you see the situation. We have to choose if we are going to trust God, or complain and fold in the midst of trials. The children of Israel complained in the midst of their test, and thus caused themselves to continue on in the wilderness for forty years. Your complaining about what you are experiencing has everything to do with your outcome. You can choose to praise God in the midst, and trust as trials come our way God will bring us through them.

Or you can complain, and not allow the patience of God to have it perfects works in you. Our affliction hasn't caught God of guard, but as trials come our way He turns them into means of blessings. Choose to thank Him instead as if it's already done, *"in all things give thanks for this is the will of God in Christ Jesus"* (1Thess. 5:18). A lot of people who knew about the diagnosis would look at me and couldn't believe it, because I never acted as if I have cancer. I didn't mope around, I chose not to speak words of defeat, and I certainly didn't look at myself as being sick.

I know there's nothing too hard for God, and I chose to rejoice and trust that. On the cancer discussion board a message came in from a guy whose dad was diagnosed with stage four pancreatic cancer. He was having a hard time dealing with it, and believed his dad was dying. I could tell he turned to the discussion board for support and comfort. We all need comforting and encouragement at times, but one lady posted, *"Just make him comfortable and reminisce with him on all the good times that you both shared."* Why would she write that, I asked myself?

Her attitude was one of defeat. We all know cancer is a serious illness, but I know a man name Jesus who can turn anything around. I wrote to him, *"Take matters into your own hands; it's not over until God says so. You guys have to fight. Get on the Internet and begin to look up natural cures for pancreatic cancer. Search out Scriptures, pray and trust God. Cancer can be reversed even in stage 4."* Please guard your ear gate, some people will think they are offering you good advice, but it could very well be the wrong advice.

One guy on the discussion board wrote to me and said, I would have to live with the disease and that cancer can't be reversed. He said that cancer basically has to be maintained and that a person could live with it and treat it, but it would never go away. Well my thoughts were, *"the devil is a liar!"* Jesus bore sickness on the cross so that I don't have to bear it. There's no way in the world I would adapt that mindset. I'm telling you the enemy will sneak in any way he can to knock you off your course.

It's during those times that you stand firm in your faith and tell the devil what the Lord said, just as Jesus did as the enemy was trying to tempt Him. When the enemy comes your way with all sorts of lies or accusations, remind him that *it is written* just as Jesus did. God's word is our most important weapon, *"For the weapons of our warfare are not carnal but mighty through God to the pulling down of strong holds; Casting down arguments, and every high thing that exalts itself against the knowledge of God"* (2Cor.10:4-5). It doesn't matter what the trial or test may be the weapons are the same; God's word, and your praise.

The thing with most people is that the enemy knows us better than we know ourselves. I don't mean for this to be a whole chapter on the enemy, because frankly he's not that important to me. It's just if I had chosen to listen to his lies I would no doubt be worse off now, than I had ever been. The lie was chemo will make you better, and after that the cancer will be all gone. But we serve a God who is certain, and His promises always come to pass. *"For all the promises of God in Him are yes, and in Him Amen to the glory of God through us"* (2 Cor. 1:20).

CHAPTER 16

Satan's Grip

When I was between the ages of eight and ten years old; I can remember going into my mother's room and kneeling by her bed and repeating the words, *"I'm dying, I'm dying, I'm dying!"* At the time I didn't realize it was the enemy, because I was so young. However, as I got older I took a look back over my life and recognized the spirit of fear, and how it had paralyzed me at an early age. I would run to the doctor about any little thing, because the enemy caused me to fear sickness. I remember one time I had a line going down the middle of my finger nail. Low and behold, I found myself running to the doctor, because I thought something was seriously wrong. Come to find out it was normal; the doctor said it was some type of pigment in my skin.

My eyes turned yellow around my pupils, by this time I'm really afraid. So there I go again, running to the doctor. Although I was diagnosed with an eye disease, it still wasn't serious. As long as I could see, I was fine. The doctor told me that my eyes are very sensitive to the UV Rays in the Sun as well as the harsh winds. He said I would have to use a certain type of eye drops and wear sunglasses. There were many other instances throughout my life that kept me running to the doctor also.

Thought I had it together

Just when I thought I had it all together, I realized I didn't. I knew that God was my Physician, and my healing would come from Him. In spite of how I felt, I chose to trust God. I talked earlier about how attitude determines outcome. Well God led me to a woman by the name of Viola. It was through her that I learned I had a long way to go. As I continued to lose weight my dress size dropped drastically. I went from a size twelve to size four in what seemed like overnight. This was very hard for me. My clothes would be so big on me that I didn't feel comfortable.

It was as if I was swallowed up by my clothes. I was shopping all the time because my weight was constantly dropping. Now I know women love to shop, but as the weight dropped, I had to shop for a different size each time, and it soon became very aggravating. I had brought summer dresses during the winter time and planned on wearing them the next summer.

Well by the time summer came around, my life had changed as well as my size. There I was with a closet full of new clothes that I couldn't wear. I had to be a blessing to someone, and give them away all except the size eight, and a few of the size ten dresses. I was determined that one day I would fit back into them. I trusted that the Lord would provide for me as I blessed someone else. After a while, I started going to consignment shops to buy clothes. It just became easier and less expensive. I would often find great deals and name brand clothes for a little of nothing and thus brought back my shopping excitement.

I thought about it, and since I had two dresses that were a size ten left, I called a good friend of mine who was a seamstress. When I got to Viola's house I told her I had been shopping so much and that I was aggravated. She saw that I had lost a lot of weight, but she thought I looked good. Every time she paid me a compliment about my size, I would put myself down. I thought that I looked like a person who smoked drugs because I was so small. I felt so skinny, and that's how I thought people saw me. My husband kept telling me that there were a lot of women who would love to be a size four.

Talking with Viola and thinking back on some of the things my husband had previously said, I realized how negative my behavior was, not concerning the illness but concerning my appearance. So I began to pray, and ask God to help me to see myself the way that He sees me, and to love myself the way He loves me. I finally realized it didn't matter how people viewed me, but how I viewed myself. Now I'm not saying that it was easy, it really was a long process. And to this day I'm still working on it, encouraging myself daily, and realizing how much God loves me.

I had to learn to love myself again. God's love is so strong, powerful, and transforming; if I could love myself with that type of love, then I would be okay. I'm not quite there yet, but I'm learning that His love doesn't just apply to Him loving us, or us loving others, but it also applies to us loving ourselves. My physical appearance had changed because of losing the weight, but love should never be based on how you or someone looks. Love is so much deeper than that. If God loved me through my imperfections, flaws and shortcomings then I could love myself.

CHAPTER 17

Deeply Encouraged

I was watching the movie Facing the Giants. I remember this one particular scene in the movie where the coach blind- folded one of the players and made him carry this kid on his back fifty yards across the finish line. The guy carrying the kid on his back started out and as time went on, the weight became heavier and heavier. The kid didn't think he could go on, but his coach kept telling him, *"Come on, you can do it. You're half way there, don't give up!"* The kid would yell, *"I can't it's too heavy, I'm tired!"* The weight will get heavy at times and even though it seems God is nowhere around, we must continue moving forward.

You will get to the end zone if you faint not. My faith was recharged. With the whole cancer situation and the choices I had to make; I thought to myself I couldn't do it, but when I looked back over the months, the thing that seemed impossible, was made possible by my faith in God.

I heard about this woman who had been battling cancer for twenty -three years. I thought to myself the pain and the weariness she must have been feeling. I had been dealing with it only several months and that was trying enough. I had heard about so many others who were battling cancer and was grief stricken. I continued to pray for others and their families, because there are so many who have lost the battle to this disease. God revealed to me that you must continue to confess the Word. Take your eyes off the situation, which I know is hard at times, and put them on God. Really believe the Word, and don't stop confessing no matter how you feel. He can't lie. Get your mind and your spirit right *"I will lift up mine eyes unto the hills, from whence cometh my help"* (Ps.121:1). Please realize your help comes from the Lord.

Like I said earlier, I sowed seeds toward my healing. I sent out prayer requests all over the world. I stayed on different Internet sites watching Benny Hinn and countless other ministries that encouraged me. People I knew were interceding for me at church, and in corporate prayer. I would call up prayer request lines and have people pray with me as well as spend time in prayer at the park.

I read about how the Lord delivered the three Hebrew boys from the fiery furnace, because they wouldn't be like everyone else and worship a golden image. They had so much confidence in God they served; they were willing to accept punishment for not bowing down to the image. God delivered them and honored their faithfulness. When we take a stand for God; whether it be doing what's right or just walking in complete faith. God honors us and will deliver us. *"Many are the afflictions of the righteous but the Lord delivers us out of them all"* (Ps. 34:19). The key word here is "all" He delivers us from ALL of our afflictions and makes them work together for the good of them that love the Lord, and are called according to His purpose.

No matter the pain I felt, I had come to believe that God had healed me. So my prayer began shift from asking for healing to thanking Him for my healing. Remember it is finished by the work that He did on the cross. Your healing was included; so began to thank Him for what He's already done. He's not going to do it again.

I dare you to create an environment of praise and thanksgiving. You'll see your spirit uplifted, you'll feel more encouraged, and the atmosphere will change. Start praying in the spirit to build your faith up and gain strength to help in your time of weakness, or doubt. Once you have begun to build yourself up in faith, you will be able to praise God in advance for the greatest outcome. Praising God is an act of faith. Basically your telling God, *"I don't know how you're going to do it, but I know You have all power, and I thank You in advance."* Believe God to the very end because your life depends upon it.

That Sneaky Devil

One day in particular I was at the office and a business partner of ours came by and handed me a book about a woman who battled cancer. I was hesitant at first to read the book, but after a couple of days I picked it up and started to look over it. As I read, to my surprise this woman had the same form of cancer as I did. We both found the lymph node in our right thigh. She had all the beliefs that I had. She did the raw foods, the diet, the exercise, and the natural supplements, just as I did. She was even out of town when she discovered something was wrong; just as I was.

Only one thing was different, and that was the way that God healed us. I believed God had healed me by the power of His Word, and my faith was strong enough that I didn't have to take chemo and radiation. Remember, we did everything the same, but she strongly advised following the treatment plans that the doctor ordered; which was chemo and radiation. She said, *"I know that you have to put all your faith in God and He is your healer, but you have to trust God to work through the doctors."* She said I should take the medicine prescribed for me lest I become worse.

Honestly it was as if God Himself was speaking to me through her book, and I began to doubt everything I believed concerning my healing. Once again fear gripped me and I spent most of that day scared and confused. By the time evening had come, I had gotten myself together. I realized that God wasn't the author of confusion and knew it had to be the enemy. I rebuked him on every hand and continued to believe God just as I had always done. The next morning my husband and I were eating breakfast with Garnell and LaShone a couple who works in the business with us. When I received a call from my sister asking me was I all right. She told me that God had awakened her around 4:00 that morning, and had her praying for me. She asked me how I was doing, as she had the sound of concern in her voice.

I really couldn't talk, because I was in front of our business partners, so I told her I would call her right back. When I called her back, I told her yesterday was a rough day for me. I told her everything I believed God was doing; I felt that He was sending me in another direction. I believed that's why God had her praying for me. I was so grateful because God loved me so much that He woke someone up on my behalf to intercede for me.

I thought that if God didn't care, He wouldn't have placed me on her heart. He would have just let me be. I thanked my sister for being obedient to His voice. God continued to show me how much He loved me, and that He was doing a great work in me for His glory. God loves us too much to leave us just as He found us. He knows exactly what our weakness and struggles are. He knows that we can't fight this battle alone and has people assisting us in the battle through prayer.

He has also assigned those who will assist you along the way. God has people who will be there to give you a word of encouragement just when you need it the most. He has that person who calls or drops by right on time asking, *"Do you need anything?"* I thank God for my friend Roxanne, even though things were rough at times we still found multiple reasons to laugh and just be silly. Talking with her made my heart glad. It allowed me for a moment to forget everything I was currently dealing with. I love this woman, and to this day, I can't remember half the things we laughed about. She was just as important to me as someone asking me did I need anything.

My husband made sure I was always okay. If he was at work, and I was having a bad day, he would immediately come home and comfort me. He made sure I had the emotional support that I needed to get through this trial. God placed a woman into my life by the name of Bonita who works in the business with us. She has a quiet spirit, and is a beautiful strong woman of God. Her personality was different from mine, but we had one thing in common, and that was Jesus. We were able to connect in the spirit as she stood in faith with me believing that God had already healed me. Whenever I had a doctor's appointment I would call her, and she would pray with me for a favorable outcome.

Even though I had gotten myself together and my faith was back on track, I told Bonita about the book I had read, and what it did to me. She began to speak words of life to me and basically told me that every situation was different, and that I have to continue to trust and believe God just as I had always done, and not lean to my own understanding. Her words were powerful and bore witness with my spirit. I was able to receive everything she said. She is just one of the many beautiful women God had placed before me, and our relationship grew from there.

Back at Dr. Yee

Time had come for another doctor's visit. I had called Emory University back to schedule a new PET and CT scan; which my husband and I said we would do in three months. We found out that my regular oncologist specialized in breast cancer, so we decided to find one who specialized in Hodgkin's disease. We had been waiting a little over a week for Emory to call back, but they never called. I assumed that maybe God closed that door, because He was going to open another door. My husband wasn't as impatient as I was, and thought that we should continue to wait for them to call.

When I walked into the cancer center, all the staff thought I looked really good. They started paying me compliments that made me feel good, especially since I had been struggling with myself image. Little did I know they were thinking I looked good for a person taking chemo. Once I got in and sat down they immediately called me back to have my blood drawn. All of a sudden this nurse came out of the blue that I had never seen before. She was kind of in a rush, as she prepared herself to draw blood from me.

She wasn't the normal person who usually drew my blood. Her first words were, *"I came to draw blood from your port."* I was thinking to myself, *"Huh!"* My husband caught on faster than I did and immediately said *"She doesn't have a port, because, she didn't do chemo."* The nurse had a look of confusion on her face and asked; *"You are Reschelle Means, aren't you?"* I told her, *"yes,* but *I didn't do chemo."* She gave my husband and I a strange look as if she was thinking, *I wish someone had told me before I got here.*

She was sent there specifically to draw blood, and as we were talking my phone started vibrating. To my surprise it was Emory University finally calling back to scheduled an appointment. I thought that was odd because I had been waiting over a week for them to call. I didn't understand what was going on, but I knew God was in the midst, and that's all I needed to know. While my husband was on the phone with Emory, I was able to get my blood drawn from my arm as I had previously done so many other times. The doctor asked me all sorts of questions like; had I been feeling well, was I having night sweats, did I had any sores in my mouth, and has my ears been hurting. I answered no to all of his questions. I can honestly say throughout this whole ordeal. I never got sick, not even once. I may have felt different pains every now and then throughout my body, but I was never physically sick not even once. That's how I know God was with me. The enemy played mind games and tried to do all he could to break me, but his tactics didn't work.

Acts of Kindness

When I found the knot and was told it was cancer, I had to withdraw from school. Mrs. Robinson, my public speaking teacher had the whole class send me cards of encouragement through the mail. The cards read things like; *"Reschelle you are a strong woman of God, and He will bring you through this. Hold on to your faith, and never doubt God."* My eyes would tear up every time I read one of those cards. Once again, God was showing me how much He loved me, and was encouraging me though their cards.

CHAPTER 18

Chemo a Huge Risk

Chemo is a huge gamble. There are no guarantees it will get all the cancer, or even if the cancer will return. Since the outcomes of the treatments were not only damaging to my body but also uncertain, I couldn't take that chance. The oncologist offers you treatments that are supposed to make you better, but most of the time, you end up a lot worse off. I know a woman who took chemo and since then has had to go to dialysis three times a week because of kidney failure. Another lady who is very dear to my heart suffers from congestive heart failure as a result of the chemo. I also know of a woman who has developed Chrome's disease because of the treatments, and another man who says his body has never functioned properly since chemo.

Seriously people, think about it; we are made in the image and likeness of God. If a little girl falls off of her bicycle and scrapes her knee. If her mother doesn't treat her knee with anything, within a couple of days it will begin to heal itself. This happens because of the laws of nature. Flowers are designed to bloom, human and animals are made to reproduce and the body is designed to heal itself. Chemo is a man invented medicine. It is not indented for the human body. It's designed as a treatment but not a cure. It cannot only target cancer cells; its toxic chemicals also destroy healthy cells. It can provide some relief for some types of cancers but the decision to do so should not be taken lightly because of the permanent damage to the body.

My Daily Regimen

I put myself on a strenuous regimen that kept me extremely busy. There were a lot of days when I was completely overwhelmed. I was taking my supplements as scheduled, exercising, drinking this mix and that one, doing everything I could to get healthy. Late one evening I had just finished washing my hair and turned the TV on. For the first time I heard a pastor by the name of Joseph Prince speak. His whole message was about grace and the Word of God began to speak through him. I was already tired of the regimen, but I was willing to do what was necessary to keep me healthy.

My regimen included:

- Rebounding (jumping on a mini trampoline) 450 jumps in the morning and 150 at night
- Taking nine natural supplements at 8:30a.m.
- A homemade fruit juice that included: apples, pineapples, grapes, strawberries, pears, and blueberries at 8:45a.m.
- Six more supplements at noon, and for lunch I would eat beans and wild rice, or I would have a salad and some almond nuts
- 2:00 p.m. a sweet potato
- 3:00 p.m. and 6:00 p.m. more natural supplements and a vegetable juice that included: broccoli, asparagus, celery, eggplant, and carrots
- 5:00 p.m. maybe a piece of grilled or baked chicken and a salad with organic, salad dressing, or beans

- Nine more supplements and my 150 rebounds at 8:00 p.m. and another vegetable juice. I also put two teaspoons of raw apple cider in my water maybe every couple of days. I drank blueberry tea, a detox tea that cleans your liver and your colon. I began to take wheat grass powder once a day around any time, aloe vera juice, and plenty of bottled purified and distilled water. I also started to take Raw Life, a green powder that has raw dried vegetables in the form of a green powder that I took several times a day. Since there was a problem with my lymphatic system, I used Lymphatonic drops several times a day in my water that promotes healthy lymphatic function
- At 9:30-10p.m. bed
- The next day I would do the same regimen all over again

This soon became a continuing headache that was hard to keep up with. My husband was spending a lot of money on supplements. I was going to the grocery store about three times a week to buy fruits and vegetables. I had to buy small amounts of fruits and vegetables because they went bad easily. It cost between $700-$900 a month to maintain and stay healthy. I'm not complaining because I was willing to do whatever it took. In my mind, the route I took was cheaper and less painful than the treatments the doctors ordered, and I am so grateful that we had the money to buy the things that I needed.

As I was watching television that evening, Pastor Prince so profoundly spoke words that set me free from the headache of the regimen. He said that we are not under the law anymore, we are under grace. The law says do, do, do and grace say it's already been supplied. What I got from that was; I had gotten so caught up with everything I had to do, to reverse the cancer, I began to crucify Christ all over again on the cross.

When Jesus said, *"It is finished"* that was it. Everything that I needed was accomplished on the cross and that included my healing. I still took my pills and did my juicing just as I had always done, but if for some reason I wasn't able to take them, I chose not to fret over it. I had to ask myself, *"do I really trust in God to heal me, or am I relying on these supplements?"* This question had me thinking.

This allowed me to know God on a completely different level. My faith was challenged and I had no choice but to grow and believe God if I was going to overcome cancer. Frances J. Roberts One Minute Meditation wrote: *"So long as there is disease in your thoughts, there will be disease in your body. Only when your mind is at rest can your body build health."* I chose to rest from it all, and examined myself to make sure, all my faith was in God.

CHAPTER 19

God Intervened

By this time it had been three months since I had my last PET scan. I had eased up on the regimen and it felt really good to be free from the schedule that I once felt bound to. However, I continued faithfully juicing several times a day and eating my vegetables. I spent every day proclaiming God's Word over my life and believing that God had healed me. Finally the moment I had been waiting for was near. I had anticipated going back, and getting the scans out of the way and returning in a week for the results.

I imagined the doctor telling me the cancer was gone. I heard about different people God had healed, people who the doctor's previously said had a certain disease, but later the disease was miraculously gone. I wanted to experience that same moment. I knew that if God could do it for those people, He could do the miraculous for me also. God had given me a glimpse that all was well, so to actually hear the doctor say the cancer was gone would be the moment of victory. Actually, the victory was the glimpse but I just needed to hear the words. God is so awesome; He will show you a glimpse of the outcome. He gives us these glimpses to keep us believing and encouraged. If it wasn't for what He showed me, my struggle could have been a lot worse than what it was.

My Neuropathy

My doctor's appointment was on a Wednesday and I had an appointment to see Terry on that Monday. When I got to Terry she began to ask me all sorts of questions. I told her all the things that I was doing, and the supplements I had been taking. She was very impressed and thought I had been doing a great job. I told her about the appointment I had on Wednesday to have my scans done over. She was excited for me and believed with me that everything would be okay. Terry had Melanoma cancer about twenty years earlier, and was cancer free also. She took no chemo or radiation. She explained how she had just come from Duke University having her scans done over and was grateful that all her tests looked good.

In a couple of days it would be my time and I was more than ready for that day to come. I wasn't quite as nervous this time as I was the last time. I had confidence in everything I had done to get me to that point; more important I had complete confidence in God.

CHAPTER 20

Back at Emory

Finally the day had come for me to be back at the hospital to have all the scans done. I woke up that morning anxious, and ready to get those tests done and over with. I thought about everything I had gone through that led me up to that point. My husband and I had to be there by 8:30 that morning. I remember thinking to myself on the way; *"Lord, it's almost over, and soon Lord, You would avenge and deliver me."* We arrived on time, and after I finished filling out my paper work they immediately called me back.

Once again I was put into this small room as the nurse inserted the same substance into my body. I drank the same liquid every thirty minutes, while they suggested I wrap myself up in a white blanket to preserve my body heat. This time my husband was allowed to sit with me. When the hour was up I had transitioned to the next room to have the scans done. Everything went well and the guy who did the scans was very nice. After everything was complete, I would have to wait till the following Wednesday for my results.

That would be my moment, the moment that everything that was wrong in my life would be right again. I wondered how the doctor would tell me, and how he would be able to explain

that the cancer was gone without the normal treatments. I had all kinds of thoughts going through my head.

In my waiting

I had finished all my appointments and all I needed to do at this point was rest in God. I would continue my daily study in God's Word and watch all kinds of inspirational TV broadcasts. I was doing my best to stay encouraged and found comfort in my family and friends. I continued to receive phone calls from people who knew about the cancer.

The more people called me, the more the enemy tried to tell me, *"You know they are only calling you, because they think you're dying."* At first I gave in to the lies of the enemy not even realizing it. I would get a little upset with people when they called, because I was starting to believe they really thought I was dying. I had to put the devil in his place once I realized what he was doing. People were calling me I hadn't heard from in years; asking me if everything was alright and some even asked to take me to lunch.

God revealed to me through a sister in Christ that I had been there for so many people, and sowed so many seeds of encouragement; that I was just reaping what I had sown. God was using others to call and encourage me as I had done so often for others. Thank you, to all who called and encouraged me during this time. Once again as I waited to return to Emory the feelings of anxiousness hit me. All I could do was continue thanking God and was eagerly waiting to share what He had done.

I know this seems crazy because I had already taken my last scans, but God was still dealing with me even up until the last hour. While I was at church one Sunday, I became very distracted. The pastor was preaching. I could see his mouth moving, but I couldn't hear anything he was saying. As I sat there, I heard the Holy Spirit tell me, *"Repeat over and over, By His stripes you are healed."* Truly my heart rejoiced when I heard those words. After all, this was one of my favorite Scriptures and one that I was very familiar with. I had already been listening to a CD from Oral Robert's ministry with so many Scriptures on it. I have to say, it was refreshing to be able to quote just one and say it over and over until I felt the power of God moving in me.

I heard Dr. Creflo Dollar speak about how it didn't take a lot of scriptures. He said to find just one and use it as your weapon. I quoted and confessed, *"By His stripes I am healed"* I said that over and over with complete assurance that God had already healed my body, and I was just waiting on the manifestation of it through the doctor's report. I woke up one Monday and I heard God say, *"Don't turn the TV on and, don't take any more supplements."* By this time I had already cut back and wasn't taking many. I paused for a second; it was no problem with the TV since I had gotten use to not having it on anyway.

With the supplements, I wanted to make sure that it was God speaking to me and not the enemy or my own thoughts. I prayed and asked God, *"If this is You speaking Lord, show me?"* and I opened my Bible to the Scripture *"Not by might nor by power but by my spirit says the Lord"* (Zech. 4:6). I said, *"Okay God I hear You."* So for the next several days I did just that. I took no supplements. I just trusted God. As I continued to believe God and thank Him for my healing the enemy wasn't letting up. When I stopped taking the supplements it seemed everything in my body began to ache.

My back began to hurt; I felt pains in my arms, and stomach. There was a sore in the inside of my mouth, and my ears were even hurting. I also had some night sweating; which are all signs of cancer. I chose not to focus on the pain because I knew it was just an illusion and that the enemy was doing anything he could to get me back on those pills, and to doubt God. I continued to quote and take God at His word. By this time I thought to myself everything that God was going to do, He was already done. The devil couldn't touch me at that point.

Some Sweet Spirited Women

One day I was at the GW Boutique and the woman who worked behind the counter was shocked to see that I had lost so much weight. I was a regular there and we frequently held conversation from time to time. As we talked, she began to ask questions about my weight. I explained to her that I had been dealing with some health issues, and had to change my eating habits. We talked about the raw food diet that I had been eating for months. She couldn't understand why anyone would want to put themselves on such a rigorous diet and asked me, *"What was wrong?"*

I told her about the diagnosis and how I decided against chemo and radiation. I began to share my faith and that I was putting my trust in God. Before I knew it, people were standing around to hear my story. I think people were just so inquisitive and couldn't understand how in the world anyone could be diagnosed with such an illness and refuse the treatments. I praise God for the opportunity to share my faith. I saw Anita there, a woman that I had met a couple years back. She and I began to talk about what had been going on with each other.

She was moved by what I had been going through and introduced me to Pam, a friend of hers who was in the store also. This was one of those days that I got up, and slipped on something to run to the store. You never know who you're going to run into. These two women had the love of God in them. They were thanking God because they had just told God they wanted to be more of a servant and help more people. Be careful what you ask for, because lo and behold they asked for someone and God sent me to them.

They were so caring and so warm. I told them that I had to be back at the doctor's office Wednesday for my results. They immediately called women together for prayer the next day. I received a text later that day with the address where we would be meeting. When I arrived, there were more women than I expected.

I started thinking to myself, *"Did they call all these women here just because of me?"* But come to find out they were already meeting for an outreach program and that's why so many women showed up. During the meeting all the women joined together in prayer for me concerning my doctor's appointment the following day.

The power of God was so real in that place. Women and children were being healed and set free that evening. I was able to take my mind off myself and look at how God was setting me up for ministry. There was a teenage girl there who suffered from migraines. I praise God for the faith to lay hands on her and believe God for her healing. Once again God showed me His love through those ladies and that was an experience I will never forget. I was introduced to some beautiful women that night, and that was an experience I will never forget.

Finally the Results

Finally the day had come. My husband and I had to be back in Atlanta by 10:30 a.m. for my results from all the scans I had done over. I woke up very anxious that morning, and anticipating the results. My husband and I had a nice drive there as we reminisced over all that we had been through. When we got there, we waited in the waiting area for almost an hour. As I sat there my heart was so heavy. The room was full of patients that were suffering from cancer. As the nurse began to call our name one by one to go, and have our blood drawn, more and more people continued to fill the room.

I saw women and men walking around with no hair. One lady was so weak I'm assuming from the chemo, all she could do was lay on the sofa; while her daughter kneeled down beside her on the floor, as they waited for their name to be called. Some of the people there looked like I did. There were young, old and all different races in one huge waiting area. Cancer is not prejudiced. It doesn't target any specific person. Anyone at anytime especially those with a history of unforgivness, bitterness, rejection, poor eating habits, and those who smoke maybe subject to this disease.

As I sat there I could only pray to myself and tell God how much I appreciate Him for not allowing me to suffer in the way that some of the other's were. After all, I hadn't done anything so great. There are so many to this day who has lost their lives to this awful disease. I'm no different than any of them. I'm sure God loved them just as He loves me. Who knows what the future holds for any of us. My advice is to always stay connected to Christ. Seek Him for who He is not just for what He can do for you. I guarantee when you begin to experience adversity, He'll already be there working on your behalf.

I urge you to understand your need for Him, and to realize that there's not ever one moment that you don't need Him. None of us deserved to be in the place that we were in. We all had different stories, different types of cancer, and we were all dealing with it in our own way. Sitting there, I could see the look on some of the loved one's faces. Some had the look of exhaustion on their faces, while I noticed one lady who couldn't stop biting her nails. What a stressful time it could be for anyone dealing with a situation of this nature. Please always pray because you never know who God has praying for you.

They finally called me back and put me in a room while my husband and I waited for the doctor to come in. My moment was finally here, where I longed to hear the words, "*The cancer is gone.*" I had visions of celebrating and calling all my friends and family. I felt so many different emotions, one of which was fear, as my husband sat cool as a cucumber. I had a Scripture in my purse. I pulled it out and began to read it silently, "*Fear not for I am with you; be not dismayed, for I am your God. I will strengthen you, yes; I will uphold you with my righteous right hand*" (Isa. 41:10). The more I read this Scripture the more peace came over me.

The doctor finally came in with a seventeen year-old intern. I was trying to read his facial expression. If he came in smiling, everything must be okay. If he had a look of dread on his face that meant something was wrong. He basically told me that my scans were fine and that they didn't look abnormal. I sat there and tried to get some understanding of what he was saying. It was if he was beating around the bush with my results. My husband began to ask him questions because he wasn't talking fast enough for us. He spoke calmly as he tried his best to explain how the cancer had disappeared, but it was obvious he didn't even know.

He said that everything looked good but they wanted to redo the scans, because the scan stopped right at my upper thigh and they wanted to get more of my lower leg on the scan. Other than that everything was okay. *"Everything looks okay"* were not the words I was looking for. I asked him, *"are you telling me there is no cancer in my body?"* He said, *"Yes, there's no cancer showing up on your scans, and everything looks clear."* By this time I was screaming, *"Yes, yes thank you Jesus, thank you Jesus!"* I was so grateful because of what God did for some of the people I knew of, He did the same for me. Everything I went though wasn't in vain.

I couldn't think by this time, but the doctor was still talking. I told him he had to talk with my husband because I was too ecstatic. I looked at the doctor, and pointed my finger toward him, and said; *"You know God did this right, God did this!"* The doctor probably thought I was crazy, but I needed him to know it was the power of God that healed me. The doctor wanted to talk more about having another scan done on my leg; as he was talking, I calmed down and started praying silently. The doctor said to my husband and I, *"Excuse me for minute"* and left the room.

He came back within five minutes and said, *"There's no need to do additional scans. We got enough of your lower leg on the scans."* However, he told me that I had to be back in three months for a follow up. If this is what the doctor ordered, I didn't mind but I chose to live by faith and the power of God that cancer shall never return! I won't live in fear that it's going to come back like the enemy wants me to. I will continue to eat right and take care of myself now that I am more educated about this disease to be able to share it with others.

Hearing the doctor say the cancer was gone was sweet melody to my ears. I looked over at my husband, who had the most beautiful and radiant smile on his face, it's one I will never forget. It was over for him as well. He showed so much compassion and was attentive during that time. We grew closer in our relationship. Our faith was challenged, but ultimately we rose to a new level in God. As we left the hospital, the song; *"In the name of Jesus, in the name of Jesus, we have the victory, in the name of Jesus, in the name of Jesus, Satan, you have to flee!"* came in my spirit.

I sung that songs for days, even as I was talking with people and telling them what God had done. Victory was won that day, and I was ready to spread the word to all who would listen, that my God is a healer. That was truly a day of triumph for my husband and I, as well as our family and friends. God showed Himself mighty that day, and for all to see and know that He is God! Before we left the doctor's office my husband had already sent a broad text telling everyone the news. When I got outside because I couldn't pick up a signal inside, I called everyone in my contact list. I had people screaming and crying with me; praising and thanking God that the cancer was gone. God showed up in power and demonstration so that all could see that there's nothing too hard for Him.

He is looking to show His power in the earth and more importantly, He's looking for someone who will believe and know that He is able. As I told my friends, they told their friends. One lady wrote me and told me she had giving her heart back to the Lord because of my story. That was confirmation that what I went through wasn't in vain. I was walking into KFC to use the restroom and there appeared to be a homeless man sitting on the curb. I was so excited and said to him. *"The doctor just told me all the cancer was gone!"* I will never forget his words, *"It sounds like the Lords doing to me."* I said, *"That's right Sir God did it, and if you believe there isn't anything He can't do for you!"*

What I learned

That evening Kerri and Quilla a couple of girlfriends of mine, we all got together for dinner to celebrate. Kerri was celebrating her divorce and Quilla was just grateful to be a part of the celebration. We all laughed, talked and had a great time. June 30 2010 is a day that I will never forget. What God did in my life was bigger than I was. God is saying; *"Be still and know that I am God."* If you're sick, first know that it's not Gods will for you to be sick. Jesus came to destroy the works of the devil. He has come to give you life more abundantly as well as good health, and by His stripes we *ARE* healed. The Scripture doesn't say, you will be healed, or you were healed, it says you are healed. I'm telling you hold on to that with every ounce of your faith, and every fiber of your being. Let God see that you trust Him. I really believe that God's wants to heal us, but sometimes it's because of our own lack of faith in His ability to do so. You know that He can do it, but you wonder if He will do it for you.

I urge you not to listen to the lies of the enemy. William Murphy said, the devil couldn't tell the truth if he wanted to. He is the father of lies. He will make everything seem worse than it really is, because the moment you allow fear in, that same moment you lose our faith. Rise up and be encouraged! Get in God's words and see what He is saying. Cancer didn't just form in my body. There were other doors that were open that allowed this disease to dwell. I dealt with anxiety and fear for many years even as a Christian.

I also struggled with forgiving myself for things from my past, and letting go of hurtful experiences. It was very important for me to recognize and ask God to heal me completely, not just my body, but my soul and emotions. Make sure your emotions are in check, and that you are whole all the way around. God is a God of wholeness and completeness. If you are holding a grudge against someone, let it go. Beverly M. Breaky wrote in her book; Choose

Life said, "Forgiveness is a state of being, not a deed." Forgiveness should be a natural part of what we do on a daily basis. You never know the things stored up in your hearts, could be the very thing that's making you sick.

Modern day physicians rarely access their patients for mental, spiritual, or emotional pain. If there is no medication to prescribe or surgery to perform, Western medicine is at a loss. Sometimes the emotional and mental pain is worse than physical sickness. That's why I needed God to heal me completely. I stop and pay attention now to how I'm feeling. I express my feeling more, and I have asked God to remove the pain of my past. My personal goals now are; to remain physically fit, eat right, stay connected to God, and to love and see myself the way God does.

I am very grateful that God has chosen me to work through.

In closing

"And they were overcome by the blood of the lamb and the word of their testimony" (Rev 12:11). Because of this Scripture, I will tell this story everywhere I go. I have peace that I am covered in His blood. I strongly advise you to keep yourself covered. His blood is His protection. Outside of His protection you're subject to anything. In the Old Testament when blood was placed over the door, the death angel would pass over it. This journey has been long, but not as long as some. God spared me for such a time as this. When the enemy tried to take me out, God said no! My heart goes out to all the families that have lost loved ones to this disease.

Just know God has someone interceding on your behalf. I'm praying like countless others for God's continual comfort and healing for you and your family. If you have been diagnosed, please remember God has the last say so. I urge you to pursue God, because in Him you will find yourself, as well as your healing. Everything isn't of the enemy. God allows certain things to come our way to see how we hold up in the midst. His purpose for our lives is greater than we can see. Faith is the key to anything you need from God. God can't lie, and His Word is proven.

I read a devotion by Sara Young that said, "*When you depend on God continually, your whole perspective changes. You see miracles happening all around, while others see only natural occurrences and coincidences. You begin each new day with joyful expectation, watching to see what He will do. You consciously live, move and have your being in Him, desiring that He lives in you, and you living in Him.*"

It is through knowing God intimately that we become like Him. This requires spending time alone with Him. Let go, relax, be still, and let God mold you. Our direction and guidance comes from Him only. The more time we spend in prayer, the less we need to seek answers from others. The only way to keep our lives in balance is to fix our eyes on Christ, and when this happen all fears and doubts are erased.

If and when you encounter a problem that you feel you have no immediate solution, either two things will happen. Either it will take you up in prayer, or down in despair. We always have a choice about how we respond to the difficulty in our lives. Our attitude is one of the main things that we can control. Be careful that you're not having a pity party while you're going through. Your attitude can either encourage others or discourage others. I knew I had a lot of people watching me. There were times I wanted to complain, and ask, "*why me?*" But I knew too many people were watching, and more importantly my faith encouraged so many others.

John Maxwell said there are two great events that happen in a person's life. One is when you are born and the other is when you find out why. I realized the thing in life that infuriates you the most, is probably the area God is going to use you in. We all must endure and stand strong as warriors, always remembering the battle is not ours but the Lords.

I prayed that if it wasn't His will that I endure certain things that He would not allow it. I did by faith stand on the Word and declare it. Sure, I did my part by eating right and exercising, but ultimately it was my faith in God's ability to heal me. If God said it in His word then I believe it, and so should you. It's that's simple. You can't please God by being fearful and doubtful. It just won't happen. You will have to pull yourself together and decide whose report you are going to believe. The battle is won first in your mind.

I had to journey along and not get caught up as to where I was going, or when I was coming out. That was up to God. *"Knowing this, that the trying of your faith, worketh patience"* (James .1:3). I had come to realize it wasn't about how long it took me to come out, it was about what was taking place on the inside of me. God was more concerned with my inner transformation than how I looked from the outside or how fast I got there. I heard a pastor say *"You can't rush God"* and that's so true. Everything has fullness of time and in that time, the very thing that you have been crying about, and up throughout the night wrestling with, God will bring it forth. Don't lose out on your blessing because of your weariness or you lack of faith.

Tremaine Hawkins has a song that says, "I Never Lost my Praise," In the midst of all life's heartache, always find a reason to praise God. Maybe you've experienced the death of a loved one, instead of being mad at God, thank Him for the time you shared with that person. I met a woman in the store who wasn't able to forgive herself, because she talked her mother into taking chemo. Her mother died during the treatments because her body wasn't strong enough to fight. This woman lived with the guilt, blaming herself for her mother's death. God used me to speak to her about forgiveness. Once she was able to forgive herself, she was able to tell God thank you and focus on the good times she and her mother shared.

It is vital that you hold on to your faith, no matter how long it takes, God is faithful. If you don't get anything else out of this book, please get that. On the days it's hard for you, start praising God by faith that He has already moved on your behalf. Praise destroys fear and the spirit of heaviness. Keep a song in your heart and praise on your lips. Believe it or not there is victory in your praise!

Thought you should know

Here is a bit of information I want you to know and understand concerning your food. Most of the time the food manufacturers and the FDA won't tell you the truth about what's in your food, because they know if you really knew what ingredients it has you probably won't purchase it.

Here's a couple of ingredients to watch out for when you're grocery shopping. If you come across these ingredients it's very important that you refrain from buying it. This could be detrimental to you and your family's health.

- Sodium Nitrates- This is a dangerous ingredient with no warnings on the label of the packaged food. This ingredient can increase the risk of cancer by 67 percent. It's a preservative found in processed meats. Sodium nitrates gives food color, adds extra flavor, preserves the meat so it won't spoil as quickly, and controls bacterial growth.
- Hydrogenated oil or vegetables oil- can cause heart disease, nutritional decencies, diabetes, cancer, as well as other health problems. It is found in sweets such as cookies, crackers, manufactured foods, and margarine. It is used to keep shelf life for a longer period of time.

- Aspartame- This ingredient causes nerve damage and can be found in diet sodas, canned foods, breakfast sausage, salad dressings, chewing gum, and Crystal Lights. This ingredient causes muscle spasms, depression, migraines, dizziness, difficulty breathing, and so many other dangerous side effects.
- High fructose corn syrup and sugar- it affects the immune system, depression, obesity, anxiety, diabetes, high blood pressure, and so many other health risk.
- White flour, artificial colors, and sweeteners should be avoided as well.

Here are a couple of spices that defend against cancer. When you're cooking replace some of the other spices with these:

- Cinnamon- lowers cholesterol
- Turmeric- this is a strong prevention against colon, breast, lung, stomach, skin, and prostate cancer
- Oregano-has a lot of antioxidants that slows down the progression of cancer
- Garlic- assist in breast cancer and kills leukemia cells
- Ginger- this helps against precancerous cells and prevents cancer causing compounds from forming in the body
- Rosemary-Reduces breast cancer by 76 percent

Some vegetables that are very healthy and high on the list to defend the body against cancer are:

- Broccoli, cauliflower, asparagus, and cabbage are especially potent against fighting cancer
- Fiber, beans, and red wine have also been known to fight cancer

- There are major benefits in consuming green tea, and blueberries and recent studies have shown that dark chocolate is beneficial also
- A plant based diet is beneficial to staying healthy and defending your body against disease

There are a lot of natural herbs and supplements you can purchase from a whole food store that you can take that will be very beneficial to you. It could be that there's some disease in your family that is genetic and you're believing that the curse has to be broken. Go ahead, get the heads up and start taking preventative measures now. The cancer in my case was reversal but maybe in your case it could be prevention. Either way knowledge is power. Get on the Internet; you will see a whole world of natural herbs and teas that are used to cure cancer, and so many other diseases.

For anyone with cancer; Essiac Tea also known as Flo Essence is extremely beneficial in fighting cancer. I recommend this tea to anyone who has cancer. It can be purchased from the whole food store.

Find Scriptures on healing, learn them, live them, believe them and begin to confess them over your life. Your mouth is a weapon against the enemy. Open up your mouth, declare and decree life abundantly, good health and break the spirit of sickness that could be hovering over you, or your loved one. If you're not used to confessions, it's a good ideas to learn more about them. Because the words you speak may be the very words that are keeping you sick. I heard a pastor preach *"Many Christians have stopped using profanity but they are still cursing."* It's something worth thinking about. Are you speaking blessings over your life, or curses?

We should be experiencing heaven right here on earth. I went through my time of suffering, now I'm rejoicing. The hedge was removed from around me, but I believe God found me to be faithful. Will he find you faithful, as you are faced with life difficulties? Are you complaining and having a pity party and turning to everyone for help, but God? I urge you to check yourself and make sure your attitude is one of gratitude the Father will be pleased with.

Whatever hurt your trials may bring, try to focus beyond the trials, to the blessings that follow. It's a blessing to be able to share your story whatever that maybe, and encourage the hearts of others. Our hurts and pain draws us closer to God; which should be our entire goal. Move forward and don't question, even as doubts may enter your mind. Chose to trust God and others will notice the light of Christ shinning upon you. Have you ever noticed during your greatest time of trials, someone will look at you and tell you that you're glowing? I've noticed that about people that I knew who were suffering, and others have told me that about myself, as I was going through trials

My last piece of advice is to stand in faith believing that God is able. *"Without faith it's impossible to please God, for he who comes to Him must believe that He is, and that He is a rewarder of them that diligently Seek Him"* (Hebrew 11:6). His healing is available to you, seek Him, cry out to Him, pursue your healing at all cost and begin to thank Him for your healing.

It's my prayer that you have come to know Christ as your personal Savior and has surrendered your heart to Him, and allowed Him to heal your mind, body and soul. I love you and may the grace of God be with you!

"What do you conspire against the Lord? He will make an utter end of it. Affliction will not rise up a second time" (Nahum 1:9).
Cancer Shall Never Return in Jesus Name!

www.ingramcontent.com/pod-product-compliance
Lightning Source LLC
Chambersburg PA
CBHW052245290526
45785CB00016B/1310